the
Macrobiotic
Approach to
Cancer

**Towards Preventing & Controlling Cancer
with Diet and Lifestyle**

the Macrobiotic Approach to Cancer

**Michio Kushi
and the East West Foundation**

 AVERY PUBLISHING GROUP INC.
Wayne, New Jersey

The medical and health procedures in this book are based on the training, personal experiences and research of the authors. Because each person and situation is unique, the editor and publisher urge the reader to check with a qualified health professional before using any procedure where there is any question as to its appropriateness.

The publisher does not advocate the use of any particular diet and exercise program, but believes the information presented in this book should be available to the public.

Because there is always some risk involved, the author and publisher are not responsible for any adverse effects or consequences resulting from the use of any of the suggestions, preparations, or procedures in this book. Please do not use the book if you are unwilling to assume the risk. Feel free to consult a physician or other qualified health professional. It is a sign of wisdom, not cowardice, to seek a second or third opinion.

Contents

Foreword

As we enter the 1980's, the East West Foundation continues to help a growing number of people secure their health and well-being. I reflected recently on this developing role as I prepared for a public lecture in Concord, Massachusetts, as a part of the Foundation's Free Library series which began earlier this year.

Over the past few years, numerous stories about the recovery of health through macrobiotics have appeared in books and magazines, and on radio and television; because of these stories, the Foundation has received thousands of letters and requests for information on the macrobiotic approach. Included in those requests have been sincere inquiries from hospital administrators and health agencies around the world.

Now, one of the most pressing needs is for institutional as well as individual training in the proper application of macrobiotic principles; and during the 1980's, macrobiotic educational activities will adapt to meet these new challenges. However, even as the scope of macrobiotics expands, it is worth keeping in mind that real change still depends on person to person communication.

Also, as we continue with a wider implementation of macrobiotic principles in society at large, the diet and way of life which provide the foundation for our health and happiness deserve our regular consideration.

As part of these efforts to improve ourselves and our world, we recommend that everyone consider the following daily reflections:

- Is my daily diet the most ideal for health and well-being?
- Do I marvel at nature?
- Do I appreciate society and all people?
- Am I grateful for life itself?

Also, in terms of daily dietary practice, please consider the following questions:

- Do I eat unrefined, whole cereal grains every day, and thoroughly chew each mouthful of food?
- Are my daily foods more natural in their quality, and do I avoid heavily processed, highly artificial foods?
- Do I use fresh vegetables every day?

- Do I season my daily meals with a moderate amount of mineral-rich sea salt rather than refined table salt?
- Do I try not to overconsume meat, eggs, cheese, poultry and other items containing plenty of saturated fat and cholesterol?
- Do I use high quality, natural grain sweetners rather than highly refined sugar or simple carbohydrates like honey and maple syrup?
- Do I avoid overconsuming fruit or fruit juices, especially those originating in the tropics?

If your answers to these questions include many "no's", we wish to suggest that you consider the dietary and way of life approach presented in this book.

This way of life, based on sound dietary practice, is being observed by hundreds of thousands of people, and is known throughout the world as "Macrobiotique," "Macrobiotica," "Makrobiotik," "Macrobiotishe," "Macrobiotico," "Makrobiotiska," "Sei-Shoku," and by many other names. Macrobiotic principles provide the focus for the educational activities of more than 500 affiliated centers throughout the U.S. and Canada, Western Europe, Central and South America, Australia, and the Far East.

Some of the benefits of eating and living macrobiotically were summed up recently by our good friend, John Denver. During a visit to Boston last month, John told us how he started macrobiotics. About one year ago, a macrobiotic friend named Ron Lemire joined John's group as a cook and masseur. As John and his group were performing on the road, Ron would prepare macrobiotic meals which everyone enjoyed very much. During these concert tours, John felt great; with plenty of energy, stamina, and mental clarity. However, after returning home, it took only several days of eating his previous diet before he started to lose his new found energy and stamina, while beginning to feel that his health was declining. After repeating this several times and reflecting on the apparent contrast in his condition, he decided to adopt macrobiotics full-time.

It is my hope that after reading this book, you will begin to understand that you too can change toward a new life of continuing health and happiness through macrobiotics.

Thank you very much.

Tim Goodwin
Vice President
East West Foundation
May, 1981

Introduction

The East West Foundation is happy to present this introductory guidebook, the *Macrobiotic Approach to Cancer*, as a part of its continuing series of publications on diet and its relationship to individual and social health.

Over the last decade, a dramatic change took place in public awareness of diet. The dimensions of this growing movement for better nutrition became apparent in 1975 when the East West Foundation, together with the *East West Journal* and other macrobiotic enterprises in Boston, sponsored the first New England symposium on macrobiotics and natural foods at Boston University. The keynote speakers at that event were Michio Kushi and Frances Moore Lappé, author of *Diet for a Small Planet*. More than 1,000 people attended, one of many indications that a growing number of people were beginning to make positive changes in their eating habits.

It was around that time that the Foundation, under Mr. Kushi's guidance, began to compile case histories and other materials on the macrobiotic approach to cancer for presentation to the general public and to leaders in the medical, scientific and governmental communities. Through these and other efforts, the Foundation has made a steady contribution toward the creation of a new international consensus with the view that diet is indeed important in the causation and prevention of degenerative illnesses such as cancer and heart disease.

By the end of the last decade, more than 18 international health agencies had issued reports linking a diet high in saturated fat, cholesterol, and refined sugar and carbohydrates with the development of many types of cancer, cardiovascular disorders, diabetes and other major illnesses. Many of these reports, including *Dietary Goals for the United States*, issued by the U.S. Senate Select Committee on Nutrition and Human Needs (which incidentally, became one of the most widely circulated documents published by the Federal Government), and the Surgeon General's *Report on Health Promotion and Disease Prevention*, suggested that many serious degenerative illnesses could be prevented simply through improvements in the daily diet. Interestingly, the macrobiotic dietary recommendations advocated over the past 25 years by Michio Kushi and his associates presaged many of the recommendations put forward in the *Dietary Goals* and similar official documents.

Much of the evidence linking diet and cancer was summarized in June 1982 in the report, *Diet, Nutrition and Cancer* issued by an expert panel of the National Academy of Sciences. "Most common cancers are potentially preventable, for they appear to be determined more by habit, diet and custom than by genetic differences," the panel concluded. Dr. Clifford Grobstein, chairman of the panel and an experimental biologist at the University of California in San Diego said, "the evidence is increasingly impressive that what we eat does affect our chances of getting cancer." He suggested that the dietary recommendations in the report, which are similar to those in *Dietary Goals*, be implemented without delay, "given the long time frame over which most cancers develop." The panel stated that the evidence it reviewed "suggests that cancers of most sites are influenced by dietary patterns."

The knowledge that diet and health are related is not new. It is fundamental to the common sense of all traditional cultures. We can trace it to the origins of modern medical practice in Hippocrates' statement that "food is the best medicine," as well to the origins of the United States in the dietary experiments conducted by several of the founding fathers, especially Benjamin Franklin and Thomas Jefferson. Jefferson felt strongly enough about the use of cereal grains as food items that he risked a severe penalty by smuggling brown rice seed out of Italy and into the Carolinas by way of France. Not only did Franklin experiment with more naturally balanced, vegetable quality diets, but he also furthered the principle of complimentary opposites—so central to the practice of macrobiotics—through his introduction of the concept of "positively charged" and "negatively charged" phenomena.

However, the founding fathers' dream of a healthy, productive and vital nation is now seriously challenged by the widespread trend toward biological and psychological degeneration that has gathered momentum in this century. Just a cursory look at the statistics reveals a frightening picture: 40 million people suffering from cardiovascular disorders; 3 million currently suffering from cancer (about 800 thousand new cases every year); over 30 million with some form of arthritis; 32 million suffering from mental disorders; 6 million suffering from alcoholism; 4 million on probation; and between 20-30 million with some form of STD (sexually transmitted disease). This trend is not limited to the United States; it can be found in one form or another in Japan, the Soviet Union, Great Britain, and in developed and undeveloped nations alike.

Fortunately, however, the role of diet in the causation and prevention of many of these problems is becoming increasingly clear and, as we proceed into the 1980's, new models of health care and social rehabilitation are emerging based on the use of diet as the major controlling factor in many disorders. Within the macrobiotic community, substantial contributions toward this effort are being made through educational programs as well as through the accumulation of case studies which point toward the use of macrobiotics in the recovery from a variety of illnesses. Moreover, a number of leading American medical centers are planning to investigate the potential of the macrobiotic approach in aiding the recovery from degenerative sickness. With heart disease for example, a controlled clinical trial, in which patients with atherosclerosis are placed on a macrobiotic diet and followed for several years, is now being planned by researchers at Harvard Medical School and one of the Harvard-affiliated hospitals. This study has the potential to produce a major impact on the current mode of treatment for heart disease.

The Foundation is pleased to offer this publication, the *Macrobiotic Approach to Cancer*, as an introductory guidebook for all those seeking information about this nutritional and way of life approach. On behalf of the Foundation, I would like to thank all of the people who contributed to this publication, including Michio Kushi, the founder and President of the East West Foundation, the Kushi Foundation, the Kushi Institute, and the *East West Journal*; Robert S. Mendelsohn, M.D., member of the Foundation's medical/scientific advisory board and well known author and syndicated columnist; Keith Block, M.D., and Penny Block, M.A., leading educators and practitioners of the macrobiotic approach in the Evanston-Chicago area; Peter Klein, M.D., a macrobiotic physician who currently resides in the Washington D.C. area; Kristen Schmidt, a registered nurse and a student at the Kushi Institute in Boston; and Marc Van Cauwenberghe, M.D., a macrobiotic physician from Ghent, Belgium, who is currently teaching at the Kushi Institute in Boston.

I would also like to thank all of those who contributed case reports for this publication, and especially Tom Monte, former associate editor of the *East West Journal* for his effort in writing several of these personal accounts.

I would also like to thank all of the people who helped to arrange the Foundation's annual conferences on the *Macrobiotic Approach to Cancer and Degenerative Disorders* from 1977-1981, including Stephen Uprichard, Tim Goodwin, Bill Tims, John Mann, Steve Gagne, Richard France, Ann Stevens La Flair, Teresa Turner and Judith Clinton, together with all of those who made presentations at these conferences, including many of the contributors to this present volume.

Edward Esko
Brookline, Massachusetts
July, 1982

CHAPTER ONE
Cancer and Modern Civilization

Michio Kushi, President, East West Foundation, Boston.
The following article is based on lectures at the Foundation's
1980 Cancer Conference and Winter 1980 Seminar.

Over the last 35 years, modern medical science has mounted a tremendous campaign in an attempt to solve the problems of cancer and other degenerative illnesses. To date, however, this large scale effort has produced no lasting, comprehensive solutions.

In the field of cancer research, for example, scientists have pioneered such techniques as surgery, radiation therapy, laser therapy, chemotherapy, hormone therapy, and others — but these treatments are, at best, successful only in achieving temporary relief of symptoms. In the majority of cases, they fail to prevent the disease from recurring, as they do not address the root cause or origin of the problem.

It is already widely known that the rates of cancer, heart, disease, diabetes, mental illness and other degenerative diseases have been steadily increasing throughout the century, and in nearly all the world's populations.[1] In fact, it is becoming apparent if this rapid expansion of biological decline continues, the civilized world may soon be threatened with widespread collapse.

We believe this collapse is not inevitable; but to prevent such a catastrophe from occuring, we must begin to approach such problems as cancer with a new orientation. Specifically, we must begin to seek out the most basic causes, and to implement the most basic solutions, rather than continue to present approach of treating each problem separately in terms of its symptoms alone.

The problem of degenerative disease affects us all in one way or another. Therefore, the responsibility of finding and implementing solutions should not be left only to those within the medical and scientific communities. It is our belief that the recovery of global health will emerge only through a cooperative effort involving people at all levels of society.

A Closer Look at Modern Civilization

The problems of cancer and other degenerative diseases cannot be separated from the problems of modern civilization as a whole. For example, I recently sat on the bench of a Boston Probate Court. It seemed that every five minutes, a different couple would enter and receive the judge's consent for a divorce. This continued throughout the day, reminding me of an automobile assembly line.

I met with several of the judges afterward and asked them why the divorce rate was increasing so rapidly. One judge answered, "We are not as respected or influential as we were in the past. At the same time, traditional values are no longer being taught in the schools, nor are they being practiced or respected at home."

---

[1]Please refer to *Cancer and Diet* (East West Foundation, 1980) for a more detailed discussion of this trend.

Everyone agreed that something should be done to prevent these disasters in family relations. One judge mentioned that in the past it was easier to guide couples in the direction of reconciliation; but lately, he went on to say, preventing a divorce had become almost impossible in most cases. Their own efforts, he said, were now directed more toward protecting the welfare of the children. They had also observed that the influence of church or school education, legal restriction or government intervention, no longer seemed capable of reversing this trend. One judge finally concluded that divorce was actually a symptom of our modern civilization itself.

The same can be said of cancer, heart disease, mental illness, and all the degenerative sicknesses. The epidemic of degenerative disease, the decline of traditional human values and the decomposition of society itself are all indications that something is deeply wrong with modern life. Let us consider the following examples:

1. A Materialistic Viewpoint.

At present, we tend to view the development of civilization in terms of our advancing material prosperity; at the same time, we tend to undervalue the development of human consciousness and spirit. But this viewpoint is out of proportion with the very nature of existence. The world of matter itself is tiny, almost insignificant, when compared to the vast currents of moving space and energy which envelop it, and out of which it has come into being.

Not only is the material world infinitesimally small by comparison, but also, as modern atomic physics has discovered, the more we analyze it and take it apart, the more we discover that it actually has no concrete existence. In other words, the search for an ultimate unit of matter, which began with Democritus' statement that reality could be divided into "atoms and space," has ended in the 20th century with the discovery that sub-atomic particles are nothing but highly charged matrixes of moving energy.

However, our limited senses easily delude us into believing that things have a fixed or unchanging quality. For example, all of the cells, tissues, skin and organs which comprise the human body are continuously changing.[2] As a result, what we think of as today's "self" is very different from yesterday's "self" and tomorrow's "self." This is obvious to parents who have watched their children grow. However, our development does not stop when we reach physical maturity: our consciousness and judgement also change and develop throughout life.

In reality, there is nothing static, fixed or permanent; yet modern people frequently adopt a more unchanging and inflexible attitude, and as a result, experience repeated frustration and disappointment when faced with the ephemerality of life. We have all heard stories about people who spent their lives gaining a fortune, only to fall into despair upon discovering that their basic needs are unfulfilled.

2. Commercialism, Artificiality, and a Decline in Quality.

Today, the successful production of consumer goods is based largely on marketing them on a mass scale. In order to succeed, a product must in some way stimulate or gratify the senses. Of itself, sensory satisfaction is not necessarily destructive. Everyone is entitled to satisfy their basic needs. However, trouble arises when sensory gratification becomes a society's driving motive. This causes a society to degen-

---

[2]For example, it has been calculated that red cells in the bloodstream live about 120 days. In order to maintain a relatively constant number of these cells, an astounding 200,000,000 new cells are created every minute, while an equal number of old cells are continuously destroyed.

erate, since the realm of the senses is so limited in comparison to our native capacities of imagination, understanding, compassion, insight, and love.

The quality of food is a good example. In the past, most people appreciated the simple, natural taste and texture of brown bread, brown rice, and other whole natural foods. Now, in order to stimulate the senses, brown rice is usually refined and polished into nutritionally deficient white rice, while whole-wheat bread has been replaced by marshmallow-soft white bread.

At the same time, a huge industry has developed to enhance sensory appeal by adding artificial colorings, flavorings, and texture agents to our daily foods. Over the last 40 years, this trend has extended to many items necessary for daily living, including clothing, housing materials, furniture, sleeping materials, kitchen utensils, and others. As many have discovered, however, the application of artificial technology to the production of consumer goods often results in a degradation in quality.

All in all, we are moving toward a totally artificial way of life, and have gotten further and further from our origins in the natural world. However, human life would not exist without the solar system or the earth, or without air, water, or vegetation. By orienting our way of life against nature, we are in effect trying to oppose and ultimately destroy ourselves.

Cancer is only one result of this total orientation. However, instead of considering the larger environmental, societal, and dietary causes of cancer, most research is presently oriented in the opposite direction; viewing the disease mainly as an isolated cellular disorder. Meanwhile, most therapies focus only on removing or destroying the cancerous tumor, while ignoring the overall bodily condition which caused it to develop.

Cancer originates long before the formation of a malignant growth, and is rooted in the quality of the external factors which we are selecting and consuming. When cancer is finally discovered, however, this external origin is often overlooked, and the disease is considered to be cured as long as the tumor or tumors have been removed or destroyed. However, since the cause has not been changed, the cancer will often return, in either the same or some other location. This is usually met by another round of treatment which again ignores the cause. This type of approach represents an often futile attempt to control only the symptoms of the disease.

In order to control cancer, we need to see beyond the immediate symptom and consider larger factors such as the patient's overall blood quality, the types of foods which have been used to create that blood quality, and the mentality and way of life which have led the patient to select those particular foods. It is also important to see beyond the individual patient and into the realm of society at large. Factors such as the orientation of the food industry, the quality of modern agriculture, and our increasingly unnatural and sedentary way of life also relate to the problem of cancer.

A Holistic Approach to Cancer

Cancer is not the result of some outside factor over which we have no control. Rather, it is simply the product of our own daily behavior, including our thinking, lifestyle and way of eating. Why is it, for example, that in considering two people, both living in the same general environment, we find that one develops cancer while the other does not? This must be the result of each person's own unique way of behavior, including all of the above factors.

When we bring these simple factors into a less extreme, more manageable balance, the symptom of cancer is no longer being created, and disappears. Accordingly, the following practices are beneficial in restoring balance to our lives:

1. Self-Reflection

Sickness is an indication that our way of life is not harmonious with the environment. Therefore, to establish genuine health, we must rethink our basic outlook on life. In one sense, sickness results largely from our arrogance in thinking that life's main purpose is to give us sensory satisfaction, emotional comfort, or material prosperity. As a result of this more limited view, we often place our happiness above that of everyone else, and our daily life frequently becomes more competitive, suspicious, and defensive; and, we continually take in more than we are able to discharge.

A more natural, harmonious balance can only be established by abandoning egocentric thinking and adopting a more universal attitude. As a first step, we can begin offering our love and care to our parents, family members, friends, and to all people in our society; even extending our love and sympathy to those we think of as our "enemies." This attitude is fundamental to the macrobiotic approach to health.[3]

2. Respect for the Natural Environment

The relation between man and nature is like that between the embryo and the placenta. The placenta nourishes, supports and sustains the developing embryo. It would be quite bizarre if the embryo were to seek to destroy this protector organism. Likewise, it is simply a matter of common sense that we should strive to preserve the integrity of the natural environment, upon which we depend for life itself. Over the last century, however, we have steadily aggravated the contamination of our soil, water and air. Is this not a self-destructive course?

Our daily way of life has also become more unnatural. Most modern people, for example, watch plenty of television, and especially color television, exposing themselves continually to great quantities of unnatural radiation. Many homes and institutional facilities also now use microwave cooking devices or electric ranges, which actually weaken our natural ability to resist disease.

Most people wear clothes made of synthetic fabrics, such as nylon stockings and undergarments, or polyester shirts. Many people also use sheets, blankets, carpets, and other household items made of synthetic materials. Synthetically produced items such as these interfere with the smooth exchange of energy between our bodies and the environment; naturally, they can also contribute to the eventual development of sickness, or make the recovery from sickness more difficult.

3. Naturally Balanced Diet

The trillions of cells which comprise the human body are created and nourished by the bloodstream. New blood cells are constantly being manufactured from the nutrients provided by our daily foods. If we eat improperly, the quality of our blood, and therefore of our cells, begins to deteriorate. Cancer, a cellular disorder,

---

[3] In a recent nine-year survey of 7,000 randomly-selected adults conducted by researchers at the Yale University School of Medicine, persons with a wide range of social contacts were found to have a better chance of leading a longer life than those with a more limited range of contacts. A solid network of friends, acquaintances and relatives was found to decrease the probability of dying by a factor of 2.3 among the men and 2.8 among the women. — From *Science News,* Vol. 118.

is largely the result of improper eating over a long period.

For restoring a sound, healthy blood and cell quality, we recommend the following dietary principles:

- **Harmony with the evolutionary order.**

When we examine characteristics such as the structure and function of our teeth or the length of the intestine and digestive tract, it is apparent that whole cereal grains comprise the most appropriate principal food for man, followed by local vegetables, beans, and other regional supplements.[4]

- **Harmony with universal dietary tradition.**

The modern diet has developed largely over the last 50 years, and includes many items which were unknown in the past such as rich, fatty foods, refined sugar and highly processed or artificial foods. At the same time, mankind's traditional staples — whole cereal grains, beans, and vegetables — are no longer consumed as principal foods. As pointed out in *Cancer and Diet,* the rising incidence of degenerative disease closely parallels these changes in the human diet.

- **Harmony with the ecological order.**

It is advisable to base our diet mostly on foods produced in the same general area in which we live. For example, a traditional people like the Eskimo base their diet mostly on animal products, and this is appropriate in a cold polar climate. However, in India and other more tropical regions, a diet based almost entirely on vegetable-quality foods is more conducive to health. When we begin to eat foods which have been imported from regions with different climatic conditions, however, a condition of chronic imbalance results, especially when we eat large quantities of sugar, pineapples, bananas, citrus and other tropical products while living in a temperate climate. Whole cereal grains, beans, local vegetables, and other regional supplements are the ideal principal foods in a temperate climate region.

- **Harmony with the changing seasons.**

A habit like eating ice cream in a heated apartment while snow is falling outside is obviously disharmonious with the seasonal order, as is consuming charcoal broiled steaks in the heat of the summer. It is better to naturally adjust the selection and preparation of daily foods to harmonize with the changing seasons. For example, in colder weather we can apply longer cooking times, while minimizing the intake of raw salad or fruit. In the summer, more lightly cooked dishes are more appropriate while the intake of animal food and heavily cooked items can be minimized.

- **Harmony with individual differences.**

Individual differences need to be considered in the selection and preparation of our daily foods, with variations according to age, sex, type of activity, occupation, original constitution and other factors. We also recommend the following daily nutritional considerations:[5]

---

[4]For a more thorough discussion of the relation of food to the process of biological evolution, please refer to the *Book of Macrobiotics: The Universal Way of Health and Happiness* by the author, published by Japan Publications, 1977.

[5]These recommendations closely parallel those made over the last five years by the Nutrition Subcommittee of the U.S. Senate, the Surgeon General of the United States, the U.S. Department of Health and Welfare, and many leading international health agencies.

1. *Water* — It is preferable to use high quality, clean natural water for cooking and drinking. Spring or well water are fine for regular use; it is best to avoid chemically treated or distilled water.
2. *Carbohydrates* — It is advisable to eat carbohydrates mostly in the form of polysaccharide glucose, such as that found in cereal grains, vegetables, and beans, while minimizing or avoiding the intake of mono- or disaccharide sugars, such as those in fruit, honey, refined sugar, and other sweeteners.
3. *Protein* — It is recommended that protein be taken primarily from vegetable sources like whole grains and bean products, while reducing the use of animal proteins.
4. *Fat* — It is better to avoid the hard, saturated fats found in most types of animal foods. High quality, unsaturated fats such as those in vegetable oils are better for regular use.
5. *Salt* — It is better to rely primarily on natural seasalt which contains a variety of trace minerals, and to avoid refined salt, which is almost 100% sodium-chloride with no trace minerals.

In a temperate, four-season climate, an optimum daily diet consists of about 50-60% whole cereal grains, 5% (one or two small bowls) of soup, preferably seasoned with miso or tamari soy sauce; 25-30% vegetables prepared in a variety of styles; and 5-10% beans and sea vegetables. Supplementary foods include occasional locally grown fruits, preferably cooked; seafood; and a variety of seeds and nuts. (A more detailed description of the standard macrobiotic diet is presented later in this chapter.)

4. An Active Daily Life

For many of us, modern life offers fewer physically and mentally challenging circumstances than in the past. As a result, functions such as the active generation of caloric and electromagnetic energy, the circulation of blood and lymph, and the activity of the digestive and nervous systems often stagnate. However, a physically and mentally active life is essential for good health. Therefore, it is advisable to supplement the more regulated patterns of modern life with regular physical and mental exercise.

Medically Terminal or Macrobiotically Hopeful?

I have met thousands of cancer patients over the last fifteen years. Of these ninety-percent or more had already received chemotherapy, radiation, or some other treatment. Many were considered terminal. In some cases there was nothing that medicine could do for them; in others, all possible treatments had already been tried, and met with no success.

Patients who have recieved treatment often take longer to recover than those who have not, and their recovery is often more complicated and difficult. With macrobiotics, we try to change the quality of the blood and cells through the most natural methods. However, when violent or artificial treatments have first been applied, a person must recover not only from the cancer, but also from the toxic and unnatural effects of the treatment.

This brings us to the difference between cases which are considered to be *medically terminal* and those which are considered *macrobiotically terminal*. A medically terminal case is one for which present treatments offer no hope of recovery. In some cases, an exploratory operation is performed and the patient is told that no treatment will be applied. Persons in this situation often have a better possibility of recovery than those who are considered hopeful and who receive radiation, chemotherapy, surgery, or some other form of treatment. A number of factors which also interfere with the natural process of recovery are summarized below:

1. Lack of Gratitude

Persons who are ungrateful frequently say things like, "Why should I eat this brown rice? Why do I have to eat these tasteless vegetables?" Or "How long do I have to stay on this diet?" An ungrateful person never thinks that he himself might have created his cancer, but usually believes instead that it is the unfair result of some unknown external factor. When someone with this attitude begins macrobiotics, they frequently return to their previous diet of meat, sugar, eggs, cheese, and other similar foods as soon as some improvement is experienced.

2. Inaccurate Dietary Practice

In some cases, the macrobiotic dietary recommendations are not well understood or carefully practiced. For example, when recommendations such as "eat 50-60% whole grains every day, prepare rice in a pressure cooker, and add a pinch of seasalt to it," are presented, most people indicate that they understand. However, upon returning home, some might cook with plenty of salt or with no salt, or with plenty of water or not enough; or they may boil or bake, rather than pressure cook. Some people might even eat 100% grain instead of 50-60%. Naturally, this type of practice hinders their recovery.

When we advise further study of macrobiotic cooking, some people reply that they already know how to cook. However, their previous style of cooking was one of the major factors which caused their cancer to develop. Persons who feel they already know how to cook often have more difficulty with macrobiotics, since they must forget their previous knowledge and start from the beginning.

3. Lack of Will

In some cases, persons who have no desire to live are introduced to macrobiotics, often by some other well-intentioned person. Persons such as this, who frequently ignore the advice they are given, have a very slight chance of recovering.

4. Lack of Family Support

Among the many patients that I have counselled were many middle-aged gentlemen who, although they were married, visited by themselves. When asked why their wives had not come, they often replied that their wives did not agree with their wish to begin macrobiotics. When asked who would cook, more often than not they replied that they would try to do it. I have also met many women who did not have the support of their husbands.

I sympathize very much with people like this, because in the real sense, they are alone. Their families lack the love and care that are essential for their recovery.

Of all the patients I have met, those who recovered were either single or had the full support of their families, even to the extent that the other family members also started macrobiotics and learned how to cook and care for the patient. Therefore, if you wish to begin macrobiotics and your husband or wife is against the idea, you might investigate the possibility of a temporary separation, at least until you recover. Someone who refuses to help their partner regain life, health, and happiness is no longer a true spouse.

5. Loss of Natural Healing Ability

Extensive chemotherapy or radiation tend to diminish the body's self-healing abilities and interfere with the natural process of recovery. If a person has completely lost their self-healing abilities through such treatments, it is doubtful that macrobiotics can help them recover.

A case can be considered macrobiotically terminal when any of these factors are present, regardless of the actual stage of the tumor. However, it is still worthwhile for persons such as this to begin macrobiotics, since it can help reduce much unnecessary pain and suffering. There have been several instances where people in terminal condition have started macrobiotics, and after several weeks became very peaceful and experienced the disappearance of pain. Then, when the end came, they were able to die in a more peaceful and dignified manner.

When a person first hears about macrobiotics, he might lack confidence in it because it seems new. If, however, he decides to pursue macrobiotics along with conventional therapy, his recovery might be slower. This approach can work temporarily, but once a patient improves, it is better to begin reducing the frequency of outside treatment. This transitional period might last from one to four months.

If surgery is considered during this transitional period, it is better to limit it to that which is absolutely necessary — for example, situations such as those in which a tumor completely blocks the passage of food through the digestive tract. Since partial blockages of the digestive vessel can be remedied through macrobiotics, surgery is advisable only in emergency situations.

Diet and the Development of Cancer

When cancer develops, a greenish shade will often appear on the skin. The appearance of this color represents a process of biological degeneration. To better understand this, let us consider the order of colors in the biological world.

Figure 1. — *The relationship between color and the development of cancer; the biological processes of humanization (I) and cell decomposition (II).*

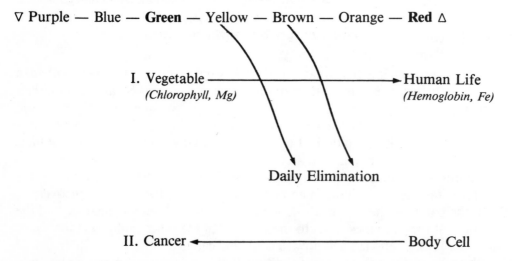

∇ Purple — Blue — **Green** — Yellow — Brown — Orange — **Red** △

I. Vegetable ⟶ Human Life
(Chlorophyll, Mg)   (Hemoglobin, Fe)

Daily Elimination

II. Cancer ⟵ Body Cell

The above diagram depicts the classification of basic colors from yang (△) to yin (∇). The process of humanization (I) represents the transformation of green vegetable life into human blood and body cells. Cancer represents a reverse process (II) in which body cells decompose, often producing a greenish shade on the skin.

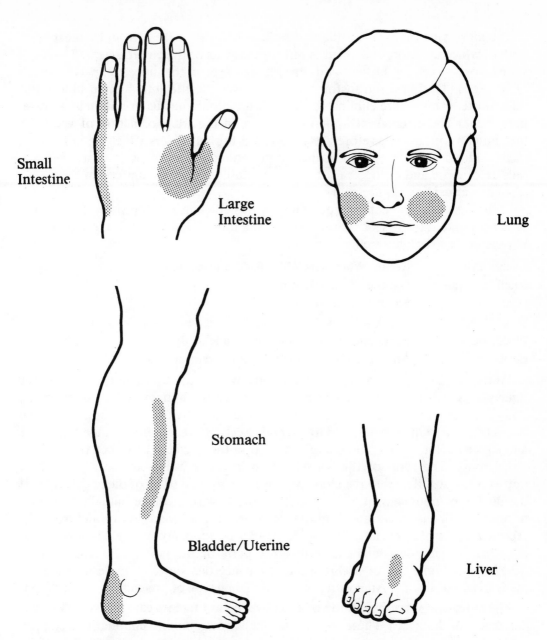

Figure 2. — *Correlations between greenish discolorations and cancer types.*

Small Intestine

Large Intestine

Lung

Stomach

Bladder/Uterine

Liver

Among the seven primary colors, red has the longest wavelength and is more yang. The opposite colors — purple, blue and green — have shorter wavelengths and are cooler. We therefore classify them as more yin.[6] Red is the color of the more yang animal kingdom, and is readily apparent in the color of the blood. On the other hand, more yin vegetables are based on green chlorophyll. Eating represents the process whereby we transform green vegetable life into red animal blood. It is based on the ability to change magnesium, which lies at the center of the chlorophyll molecule, into iron, the element which forms the basis of hemoglobin.

[6]For an explanation of the principles of yin and yang, please refer to the *Book of Macrobiotics* by the author, published by Japan Publications.

The more yin colors — purple and blue — appear in the sky and atmosphere; both of which are more expanded or yin components of the environment. The more yang colors — yellow, brown, and orange — appear in the more compacted world of minerals. During the transformation of vegetable life into human blood and cells, waste products are eliminated through functions such as urination and bowel movement. These represent in-between stages in the transformation of vegetable into human life, and therefore are yellow and brown, colors which lie in between green and red in the spectrum. Cancer represents a reverse process in which body cells decompose and change back toward vegetable life, and manifests in the greenish shade appearing on the skin.

In the case of colon cancer, for example, this color might appear on the outside of either hand in the indented area between the thumb and forefinger (see figure 2). Several other examples are listed below:[7]

Cancer Type	Region Where Greenish Shade Might Appear
Small Intestine	Outside of the little finger
Lung	Either or both cheeks
Stomach	Along the outside front of either leg, especially below the knee
Bladder/Uterine	Around either ankle on the outside of the leg
Liver	Around the top of the foot in the central area

To further understand how cancer develops, we can use the analogy of a tree (see figure 3). A tree has structure which is opposite to the human body. For example, body cells have a more closed structure and are nourished by red blood, while the leaves of a tree, which correspond to the body's cells, have a more expanded structure and a green color. A tree's lifeblood comes from the nutrients absorbed through external roots. The roots of the body lie deep in the intestines in the region where nutrients are absorbed into the blood and then distributed to all of the body's cells. If the quality of nourishment is chronically poor, however, cells eventually lose their normal functional ability and begin to deteriorate. This condition results from the repeated intake of poor nutrients and does not arise suddenly. While it is developing, many other symptoms might arise in other parts of the body. Therefore, cancer develops over time out of a chronically pre-cancerous state. In my estimation, as many as 80-90% of the American people have some type of pre-cancerous condition.

The repeated overconsumption of excessive dietary factors causes a variety of adjustment mechanisms. These include normal functions like elimination, respiration, and others, as well as the chronic discharge and pre-cancerous storage of excess. Several of these processes are outlined below:

1. Normal Discharge
If we eat a reasonable volume of high quality food and maintain an active daily life, normal biological functions — urination, bowel movements, respiration, perspiration, etc. — efficiently discharge any excess. Discharge also takes place through daily thinking and activity, as well as through normal functions like menstruation, childbirth, and lactation.

2. Abnormal Discharge
However, practically everyone eats and drinks excessively, and this often triggers a

---

[7] For additional correlations, please refer to *Natural Healing through Macrobiotics* and *How to See Your Health: the Book of Oriental Diagnosis* by the author, published by Japan Publications.

variey of abnormal discharge mechanisms such as diarrhea, overly frequent bowel movements, or frequent urination beyond the normal 3-4 times per day. Habits like scratching the head, tapping the feet, frequent blinking, and others also represent abnormal discharges, as do emotions such as anger. Periodically, excess is discharged through more acute or violent symptoms such as a sudden fever, coughing, or sneezing.

3. Chronic Discharge

Chronic discharges are the next stage in this process and often take the form of skin diseases. These are common in cases where the kidneys have lost their ability to properly cleanse the bloodstream. For example, skin markings such as freckles and dark spots indicate the chronic discharge of sugar and other simple carbohydrates; while white patches indicate the discharge of milk, cottage cheese, and other dairy products.

Hard, dry skin arises after the bloodstream fills with fat and oil, eventually causing blockage of the pores, hair follicles, and sweat glands. When these blockages

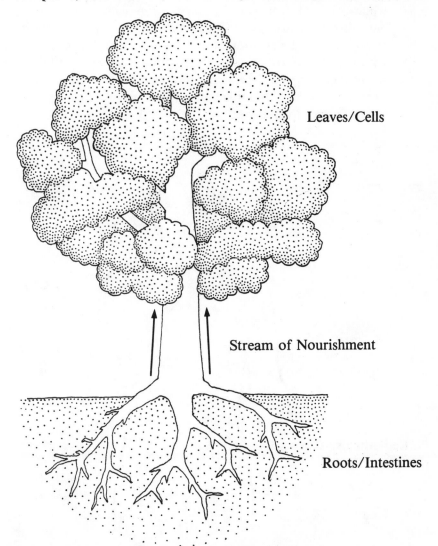

Leaves/Cells

Stream of Nourishment

Roots/Intestines

Figure 3. — *Comparison between a tree and the human body.*

prevent the flow of liquid toward the surface, the skin becomes dry. Many people believe that this condition results from a lack of oil, when in fact it is caused by the intake of too much fat and oil.

4. Accumulation

If we continue to eat poorly, we eventually exhaust the body's ability to discharge. This can be serious if an underlying layer of fat has developed under the skin which prevents discharge toward the surface of the body. This condition is caused by the repeated overconsumption of milk, cheese, eggs, and other fatty, oily, or greasy foods.

When this stage has been reached, internal deposits of mucus or fat begin to form, initially in areas which have some direct access to the outside. These deposits frequently develop in the following regions (see figure 4):

1. *Sinuses* — The sinuses are a frequent site of mucus accumulation, and symptoms such as allergies, hay fever, and blocked sinuses often result. Hay fever and sneezing arise when dust or pollen stimulate the discharge of this excess, while calcified stones often form deep within the sinuses. Thick, heavy deposits of mucus in the sinuses diminish our mental clarity and alertness.

2. *Inner Ear* — The accumulation of mucus and fat in the inner ear interferes with the smooth functioning of the inner ear mechanism and can lead to frequent pain, impaired hearing, and even deafness. About 12 million Americans are now deaf, and this number is steadily increasing, while millions more suffer from impaired hearing.

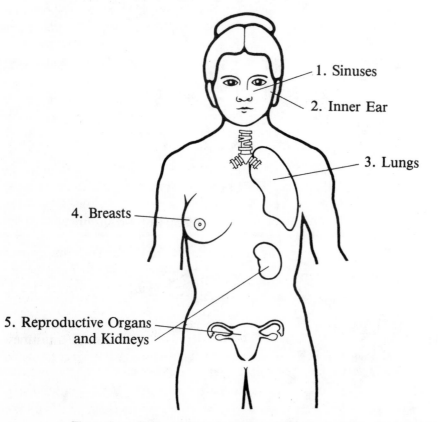

Figure 4. — *Frequent sites of mucus and fat accumulations in the body.*

3. *Lungs* — Various forms of excess often accumulate in the lungs. Aside from the obvious symptoms of coughing and chest congestion, mucus often fills the alveoli, or air sacs, and breathing becomes more difficult. Occasionally, a coat of mucus in the bronchi can be loosened and discharged by coughing, but once the sacs are surrounded, it becomes more firmly lodged and can remain there for years. Then, if air pollutants or cigarette smoke enter the lungs, their heavier components are attracted to and remain in this sticky environment. In severe cases these deposits can trigger the development of lung cancer. However, the underlying cause of this condition is the accumulation of sticky fat and mucus in the alveoli and in the blood and capillaries which surround them.

4. *Breasts* — The accumulation of excess in this region often results in a hardening of the breasts and the formulation of cysts. Excess usually accumulates here in the form of mucus and deposits of fatty acid, both of which take the form of a sticky or heavy liquid. These deposits develop into cysts in the same way that water solidifies into ice, and this process is accelerated by the intake of ice cream, cold milk, soft drinks, orange juice, and similar foods which produce a cooling or freezing effect.

   Women who have breastfed are less likely to develop breast cysts or cancer. Women who do not nurse miss this opportunity to discharge through the breasts, and therefore face a greater possibility of excess accumulating in this region.

5. *Reproductive Organs and Kidneys* — The prostate gland is a frequent site of accumulation. As a result, it often becomes enlarged, and hard fat deposits or cysts often form within and around it. This is one of the principal causes of impotency.

   Since the female reproductive organs connect to the outside, excess also accumulates there. This can lead to the formation of ovarian cysts as well as the blockage of the Fallopian tubes. In many cases, mucus or fat in the ovaries or Fallopian tubes prevents the passage of the egg and sperm, resulting in an inability to conceive.

   As a result, many women suffer from chronic vaginal discharge. Problems with the female sexual organs have become so widespread in America that, in a recent survey, 50% of all American women were found to have had a hysterectomy by the age of 60.

   Deposits of mucus and fat also accumulate in the kidneys. Problems arise when these elements clog the fine network of cells in the interior of these organs, causing them to accumulate water and become chronically swollen. Since elimination is hampered, fluid which cannot be discharged is often deposited in the legs, producing periodic swelling and weakness. If someone with this condition consumes a large quantity of foods which produce a chilling effect, the deposited fat and mucus will often crystallize into kidney stones.

Although these symptoms seem unrelated, they all stem from the same underlying cause. However, modern medicine often does not view them as such. For example, when someone with hearing trouble or cataracts visits a hospital, they are often referred to an ear or eye specialist. However, a symptom such as cataracts indicates a variety of related problems, such as mucus accumulation in the breasts, kidneys, and sexual organs.

If, beyond this point, a person continues to eat excessively, the deeper internal organs start to be affected. One common example is the accumulation of cholesterol and saturated fat in and around the heart and in the arteries. If a person reaches the stage where all of the major organs contain heavy deposits, while discharge through the skin is blocked by a layer of fat, obesity and toxic, acidic blood often result.

An organism cannot survive in this condition. Therefore, in order to prevent immediate collapse, toxins are localized, leading to the formation of a degenerative quality cell. As long as improper nourishment is taken in, the body will continue localizing toxins, resulting in the continual growth of the cancer. When a particular location can no longer absorb toxic excess, the body must search for another place to localize it, and so the cancer spreads. This continues until the cancer spreads throughout the body and the person eventually dies.

Therefore, symptoms like vaginal discharges, ovarian cysts, hardening of the breasts, skin discharges, dry skin, and similar problems all represent pre-cancerous conditions. However, they need not develop toward cancer if we change our way of eating.

Diagnosing Pre-Cancerous Conditions

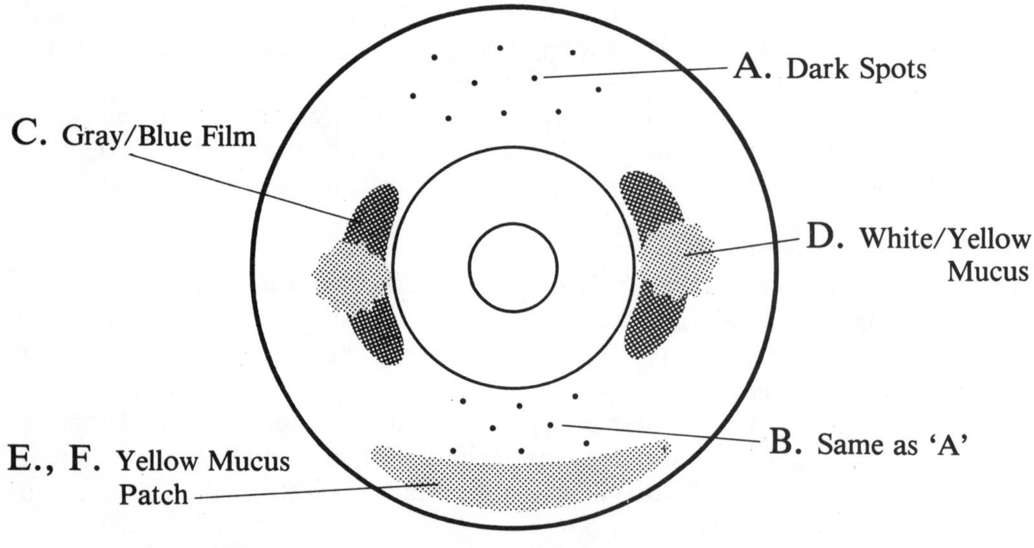

Figure 5. — *Eye-white markings.*

Pre-cancerous conditions can be diagnosed through careful observation of the eye-whites.[8] Pre-cancerous conditions often correlate with the following markings:

    A. *Calcified deposits in the sinuses* are frequently indicated by dark spots in the upper portion of the eye-white.

    B. *Kidney stones and ovarian cysts* are often indicated by dark spots in the lower eye-white.

    C.,D. *The accumulation of mucus and fat in the centrally located organs (liver, gallbladder, spleen, and pancreas)* frequently appears in the form of a blue,

---

[8]For a more thorough explanation of this and other traditional methods of diagnosis, refer to *How to See Your Health: the Book of Oriental Diagnosis* by the author.

green, or brownish shade, or white patches, in the eye-white on either side of the iris. This often indicates a reduced functioning in these organs.

E. *Accumulations of fat and mucus in and around the prostate* are often indicated by a yellow coating on the lower part of the eyeball.

F. *Fat and mucus accumulations in the female sex organs* are frequently indicated by a yellow coating in the same area of the eye as E above. Vaginal discharges, ovarian cysts, fibroid tumors, and similar disorders are also possibly indicated.

Yin and Yang in the Development of Cancer

Yin and yang refer to the two primary forces or tendencies which exist throughout the universe. In the human body, for example, the two branches of the autonomic nervous system — the ortho-sympathetic and para-sympathetic — work in an antagonistic, yet complementary manner to control the body's automatic functions. The endocrine system functions in a similar way. The pancreas, for example, secretes insulin, which controls the blood sugar level, and also secretes anti-insulin, which causes it to rise.

Among sicknesses, some are caused by an overly expanding tendency; others result from an overly overly contracting tendency, while others result from an excessive combination of both. In the Orient, the more expanding tendency is referred to as *yin*; while the opposite, more consolidating tendency is called *yang*.[9]

An example of a more yang sickness is a headache caused when the tissues and cells of the brain contract and press against each other, resulting in pain; while a more yin headache arises when the tissues and cells press against each other as the result of swelling or expansion. Therefore, similar symptoms can arise from opposite causes.

Epilepsy is a more yin disorder caused by the overconsumption of soda, fruit juice, coffee, and other liquids, as well as sugar and other foods which turn into liquid after being eaten. This disorder can be readily controlled by eliminating or minimizing the intake of these items.[10]

Cancer is characterized by a rapid increase in the number of cells, and in this respect, is a more expansive or yin phenomenon. However, the cause of cancer is more complex. As everyone knows, cancer can appear almost anywhere in the body. Skin, brain, liver, uterine, colon, lung, and bone cancer are just a few of the more common types. Each type has a slightly different cause.

To better understand this, let us consider the difference between prostate and breast cancer, both of which are increasing in incidence. Recently, female hormones have been used to temporarily control prostate cancer. At the same time, a male hormone has been found to have a similar controlling effect with breast cancer.

---

[9]The terms "yin" and "yang" ("Yo" in Japanese) have been used commonly in the Orient for thousands of years. For example, the terms *Yin-Kyoku* and *Yo-Kyoku* are frequently used in the modern study of electricity and magnetism to describe a negative and a positive charge or magnetic pole. At the same time, an electron is called *Yin-Denshi*, or "yin electric particle," and a proton is called *Yo-Denshi*, or "yang particle." These terms are used frequently in daily conversation.

[10]An example of physiological changes which occur from alterations in yin and yang balance can be seen in the phenomenon known as *hemolysis*. When red blood cells are placed in water (more yin), they swell and finally burst. If they are placed in a 0.9% saline solution (more balanced), they remain unchanged, since the concentration of salt in the solution is about the same as the total concentration of salts in the blood plasma and in the red cell itself. If red cells are placed in a more concentrated (yang) solution, for example, 2% salt, water begins to leave the cells and they shrink and shrivel.

Suppose, however, that female hormones were given to women with breast cancer. This would cause their cancers to develop more rapidly, while male hormones would accelerate the growth of prostate cancer. Therefore, women who have taken birth control pills containing estrogen have a higher risk of developing breast cancer.

As we can see in the above example, breast and prostate cancer have opposite causes. Since more yin female hormones help neutralize prostate cancer, we can assume that this condition is caused by an excess of yang factors. Since breast cancer can be temporarily neutralized by more yang male hormones, this disorder has an opposite, or more yin, cause. Cancers of the stomach, esophagus, and mouth are similar to breast cancer in that their primary cause is an excess of more yin factors, while cancers of the lower digestive tract are generally caused by excess of more yang factors, as is prostate cancer.

In general, more yin cancers are accelerated by the intake of more yin or expansive foods such as sugar, fruit, dairy products (especially milk and light cheese), oil, flour (especially white flour), alcohol, drugs, coffee, honey, maple sugar and other sweets, chemicals, potatoes, tomatoes, and spices and stimulants. On the other hand, more yang cancers are accelerated by the repeated overconsumption of more yang or contractive foods including meat, salt, eggs, hard salty cheeses, poultry, and fish.

The Japanese tend to develop more stomach cancers because they eat a large volume of sugar, chemicals, and more yin, chemically grown and treated white rice. Americans develop more colon cancers largely because of a high intake of meat, eggs and other more yang items. Of course, yin and yang foods are always eaten in combination. But certain people eat a larger volume of one, while some eat a larger volume of the other. A woman develops breast cancer largely through the overconsumption of more yin foods, especially milk, sugar, fruit, and fruit juice; while prostate cancer develops largely from the excessive intake of eggs, meat, salty cheese, poultry, and other more yang items.

To summarize, some cancers can result from an excess of more extremely yin foods, others from an excess of more extremely yang items, and others from an excess of both extremes. A chart listing common varieties of cancer and their classification according to yin and yang is presented below:

General Yin and Yang Classification of Cancer Sites

More *Yin* Cause	More *Yang* Cause	*Yin* and *Yang* Combined
Breast	Colon	Lung
Stomach	Prostate	Bladder
Skin	Rectum	Uterus
Mouth (except tongue)	Ovary	Kidney
Esophagus	Bone	Spleen
Leukemia	Pancreas	Melanoma
Hodgkin's Disease	Brain (inner regions)	Tongue
Brain (outer regions)		

What are known as carcinogenic factors can also be understood in terms of yin and yang. For example, a number of years ago, tar was suspected as a cancer-causing agent. In order to prove this hypothesis, a group of Japanese scientists repeatedly applied tar to the ears of rabbits. After many days of continued application, cancer started to develop, and it was decided that tar must be a carcinogenic agent. However, tar is not in and of itself a cancer causing factor. Tar is a more condensed or yang compound. By continuously applying a more yang factor such as this to the rabbits' skin, the cells became inflamed by drawing yin factors from the bloodstream and started to spread. This is simply an illustration of the natural law "at the extreme, yang produces yin; while at the extreme, yin will also produce yang."[11]

Similarly, the sun has often been accused of causing skin cancer. However, of itself, the sun is not the cause of this disorder. Repeated exposure to a more yang factor, such as the sun, might trigger a proliferation of cells, especially when foods such as oil, fat, sugar, milk, Coca-Cola, and other extremely yin items are eaten daily. These foods provide the underlying basis for skin cancer, a more yin disorder, to develop, the yang factor of sunlight serves only as a catalyst to localize these factors on the skin.

Several years ago it was discovered that the fat and protein molecules contained in grilled meat or fish often change into cancerous cells. However, people have eaten foods such as grilled sardines, fish, or meat for thousands of years, yet rarely developed cancer. Traditionally, these foods were eaten together with plenty of fresh green vegetables, creating a complementary balance which prevented cancer from developing.

The Standard Macrobiotic Diet

To help offset the development of cancer, it is important to recover a more moderate balance in the daily diet. A more centrally-balanced diet based on foods

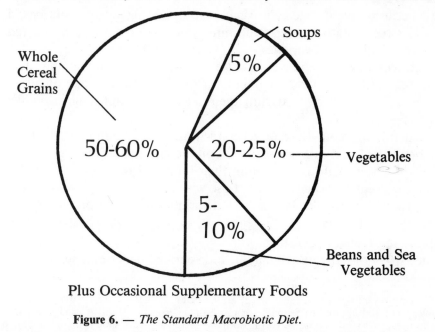

Figure 6. — *The Standard Macrobiotic Diet.*

---

[11]Another familiar example is the activation and subsequent expansion (yin) of atoms and molecules following exposure to heat (yang). The slowing down and subsequent condensation (yang) of atoms and molecules following exposure to cold (yin) also illustrates this basic principle.

such as whole cereal grains, beans, and cooked vegetables can therefore support the recovery from both more yin and more yang cancers (see figure 6).

This does not mean, however, that the same dietary program should be adopted in every case. Various adjustments are advisable in every circumstance. Before considering these adjustments, however, let us first review the centrally balanced, standard macrobiotic diet. Please keep in mind that these guidelines do not represent medical advice, and are not intended to replace personal study with a qualified macrobiotic advisor.

1. Whole Cereal Grains

We recommend that whole cereal grains comprise 50-60% of the volume of every meal. Whole grains include brown rice, millet, whole wheat, oats, rye, corn, barley, and buckwheat. Please note that whole grains are preferable to flour products, as flour products tend to be more difficult to digest and can be mucus producing.

2. Soup

One or two cups or small bowls of soup may be included in the daily diet, especially those seasoned with *miso* or *tamari* soy sauce.[12] We recommend that soup not taste overly salty, and include a variety of suitable vegetables. Wakame seaweed can also be included on a daily basis. Soups made with whole grains and beans can also be served from time to time.

3. Vegetable Dishes

Vegetable dishes may comprise 25-30% of daily intake. Vegetables for daily use include green cabbage, kale, Swiss chard, watercress, Chinese cabbage, bok choy, dandelion, burdock root, carrots, daikon radish, turnips, and their green tops, onions, acorn, Hubbard, and butternut squash, radish, cauliflower, and other locally available varieties.

It is better to avoid vegetables such as tomatoes, eggplant, potatoes, asparagus, spinach, sweet potatoes, beets, zucchini, yams, avocado, green and red peppers, and other highly acidic varieties.

Vegetables may be prepared in a variety of ways, including boiling, steaming, and sauteeing. Persons with cancer might wish to limit their intake of oil by avoiding deep-fried foods, and by restricting their use of oil in sauteeing vegetables to about twice per week.

In general, up to one-third of vegetable intake may be eaten in the form of salad. (It is better to avoid mayonnaise and commercial salad dressings.) However, persons with cancer might need to limit their intake of raw salad. A small volume of salad may be eaten on occasion by those with more yang types of cancer, while it is not advisable for persons with more yin varieties of cancer or cancers caused by an excess of both factors.

4. Beans and Sea Vegetables

About 5-10% of daily intake may include cooked beans and sea vegetables. How-

---

[12]*Miso* is processed from soybeans, cereal grains (such as barley, rice or wheat) and sea-salt. It is naturally aged and allowed to ferment for more than 1½ years. *Miso* is used in a paste form, and *tamari* soy sauce is used in a liquid form. Both are processed from similar ingredients, and have been used for many centuries throughout the Orient. In traditional usage, "tamari" means the thick liquid squeezed from fermented miso, but in macrobiotics it is used to distinguish traditionally processed, natural soy sauce from commercially available varieties which are artificially processed. Both miso and tamari are available in most natural food stores.

ever, since beans in general contain plenty of fat and protein, it is advisable for persons with cancer to eat a small volume while limiting their intake to varieties which are lower in fat such as azuki beans, chickpeas, and lentils.

Mineral-rich sea vegetables can be used on a daily basis in soups, with beans, or as side dishes. Sea vegetables such as hiziki, kombu, wakame, nori, dulse, and Irish moss are fine for regular use.

5. Supplementary Foods

Persons in good health may wish to include additional supplementary foods. Among these, a small volume of white meat fish may be eaten once or twice per week. White meat fishes generally contain less fat than red meat or blue skin varieties. A small volume of fruit dessert, as well as some fresh and dried fruit, may also be eaten on occasion. It is advisable to eat only locally grown fruits. Thus, if you live in a temperate zone, avoid tropical and semi-tropical fruit (oranges, bananas, pineapples, etc.) It is generally advisable to limit fruit intake to several times per week, while snacks made from roasted seeds, grains or beans, lightly seasoned with tamari, may be enjoyed from time to time.

6. Beverages

Recommended daily beverages include roasted bancha (kukicha) twig tea, roasted brown rice tea, roasted barley tea, dandelion tea, and cereal grain coffee. Any traditional tea that does not have an aromatic fragrance or a stimulant effect can also be used.

7. Additional Suggestions

- *Cooking oil.* If you wish to improve your health, use only high-quality sesame or corn oil in moderate amounts.
- *Salt.* Naturally processed, mineral rich sea salt and traditional, non-chemicalized miso and tamari soy sauce may be used as seasonings. It is recommended that daily meals not have an overly salty flavor.
- The following *condiments* are also recommended for regular use:
  - *Gomasio* (sesame salt) - 10 to 12 parts roasted sesame seeds to 1 part sea salt ground together in a small earthenware bowl called a *suribachi.*
  - *Roasted kombu or wakame powder* - Bake kombu or wakame in the oven until black. Crush in a *suribachi* and store in a jar or small container.
  - *Umeboshi plum*[13]
  - *Tekka*[14]
  - *Tamari* soy sauce (moderate use only)
- You may eat regularly 2-3 times per day, as much as you want, provided that the proportion is correct and chewing is thorough. Please avoid eating for approximately 3 hours before sleeping. For thirst, use any of the beverages mentioned previously or drink small amounts of water (preferably spring water) which is not icy cold.

---

[13]Plums which have been dried and pickled for many months with sea salt are called *ume* (plum) -*boshi (dry) in Japanese. Shiso* (Beefsteak) leaves are usually added to the plums during pickling to impart a reddish color and natural flavoring. Umeboshi plums stimulate the appetite and digestion, and aid in maintaining an alkaline blood quality. They are available in many natural food stores.

[14]Tekka is literally translated as "iron-fire" [from the Japanese *tetsu* (iron) and *ka* (fire).] This traditional condiment is made from carrot, burdock and lotus root which have been finely chopped and sauteed in sesame oil and miso for many hours. Tekka is usually prepared in a cast iron pan. It is available in many natural food stores.

Guidelines for Adjusting the Standard Diet

When properly applied, the standard macrobiotic diet can help to restore an excessively yin or yang condition to one of more natural balance. However, slight modifications are needed in every case. A few sample modifications for more yin or more yang varieties of cancer are presented below:

More Yin Cancer	Food	More Yang Cancer
Minimize use of corn.	*Grains*	Avoid buckwheat.
Stronger flavor (more miso or tamari).	*Soup*	Milder flavor (less miso or tamari).
Greater emphasis on root varieties (burdock, carrot, turnip, etc.)	*Vegetables*	Greater emphasis on leafy green varieties daikon, carrot, or turnip greens, kale, watercress, etc.
Stronger seasoning (miso, tamari, sea salt); slightly heavier cooking.		Milder seasoning; more light cooking.
More strongly seasoned; use less often.	*Beans*	More lightly seasoned; may use regularly.
Avoid completely.	*Fruit dessert*	Small amounts of cooked seasonal fruit only when craved.

Because of the differences in cause, no single approach is beneficial for all cancers. For example, there are several clinics in Texas, Southern California and Mexico which recommend a diet of raw salads, fruit, and other more yin items for all types of cancer. In some cases, an approach such as this can help offset more yang types of cancer. But if a person with more yin cancer were to eat a diet such as this, the results could be disastrous.

If you are generally healthy, fish and fruit desserts can be eaten on occasion. However, it is better for persons with more yin cancers to avoid fruit completely — even cooked apples and other more yang fruits. Persons with more yang cancers may occasionally have small amounts but only when craved. On the other hand, it is better for persons with more yang cancers to stay away entirely from all animal food, relying only on more lightly cooked vegetable-quality foods. It is also recommended that persons with cancer avoid nuts and nut butters which are very oily and high in protein.

Special Dishes and Considerations

Below are several adjustments which are advisable when preparing and using condiments and other foods:

• **Gomasio.** *For more yin cancer:* Prepare with 10-12 parts roasted sesame seeds to 1 part salt. *For more yang cancer:* Prepare with 14-16 parts roasted sesame seeds to 1 part salt. *For cancers caused by a combination of both:* Prepare with 12 parts seeds to 1 part salt. Use about one teaspoonful per day.

• **Roasted Seaweed Powder.** *For more yin cancer:* Can be used more frequently in larger amounts (approximately 1 teaspoonful per day). *For more yang cancer.* Slightly less volume is advisable (approximately ½ teaspoonful per day). *For* *cancers caused by a combination of both:* An in-between volume is recommended (½-1 teaspoonful per day).

•**Umeboshi Plum.** Can be used by persons with all types of cancer. Umeboshi plums contain a harmonious balance of more yin factors, such as the natural sourness of the plum, and more yang factors created by the salt, pressure, and aging used in their preparation.

•**Tekka.** This more yang condiment can be used by persons with all types of cancer. *For more yin cancer:* Can be used every day (approximately ½ teaspoonful). *For more yang cancer:* It is advisable to use small volume only on occasion.

•**Tamari-Nori Condiment.** This special condiment, made with nori seaweed, can be used to help the body recover its ability to discharge toxic excess. To prepare:
1. Place several sheets of nori in water (about ½ cup) and simmer until most of the water cooks down to a thick paste.
2. Add tamari soy sauce several minutes before the end of cooking for a light to moderate taste.

This condiment can be eaten by persons with all types of cancer. *Those with more yang cancer* may use a slightly smaller volume (for example ½ teaspoonful per day) while *those with more yin cancer* may use up to 1 teaspoonful per day. *Those with cancers caused by a combination of both* may eat an in-between volume.

•**Shio-Kombu Condiment.** This more yang condiment is very rich in minerals and aids in the discharge of toxins. To prepare:
1. Soak kombu until soft and then chop into one-inch square pieces.
2. Add sliced kombu (about 1 cup) to ½ cup of water and ½ cup of tamari soy sauce.
3. Bring to a boil and simmer until the liquid evaporates.
4. Place in a covered jar to keep for several days.

Several pieces of shio-kombu may be eaten on a daily basis.

•**Bancha Tea.** There are now several varieties of bancha tea presently available, including *green tea,* usual *bancha tea,* and *bancha stem tea.* All are produced from the same tea bush. Green tea is harvested in the summer and consists of the green leaves taken from the upper parts of the bush. However, some leaves are left on the plant until fall, at which time they become harder, drier, and brownish in color. These leaves are used to produce usual bancha tea. Bancha stem tea is made from the branches and stems of the plant which are dry roasted. More yin green tea contains plenty of vitamin C and can be used to help offset the toxic effects resulting from the overconsumption of animal foods, while more yang bancha stem tea contains less vitamin C but plenty of calcium and minerals. It is advisable for all cancer patients to use the bancha stem tea as their main beverage. However, persons with more yang cancers may occasionally use the green tea for a short duration only. Green tea is not recommended for persons with other types of cancer.

- **Nishime (Waterless Cooking) Dish.** This special method of preparing vegetables is helpful in restoring strength and vitality to someone who has become physically weak. To prepare:
  1. Use a heavy pot with a heavy lid.
  2. Soak kombu until soft and cut into one-inch square pieces.
  3. Place kombu in bottom of pot and add just water enough to cover.
  4. Add chopped carrots, daikon, turnip, or burdock root, lotus root, onions, hard winter squash (acorn or butternut), and cabbage. These should be cut into 2-inch chunks and layered on top of the kombu.
  5. Sprinkle small volume of sea salt over the vegetables.
  6. Cover and set flame to high until a high steam is generated. Lower flame and cook 15-20 minutes in the high steam. If water evaporates during cooking, add more to the bottom of the pot.
  7. When each vegetable has become soft and edible, add tamari soy sauce and mix the vegetables by shaking the pot.
  8. Replace cover and cook over a low flame for two minutes.
  9. Remove cover, turn off the flame, and let the vegetables sit for about two minutes, allowing all the steam to escape. There should be no water left in the bottom of the pot.

  It is recommended that this dish be included anywhere from 2-4 times per week.

- **Steamed Greens Dish.** To prepare:
  1. Wash and slice the green leafy tops of vegetables such as turnip, daikon and carrots. (Kale, watercress, or Chinese cabbage may also be used.)
  2 . Place cut vegetables in a small amount of water at a high boil.
  3 . Cover and steam for seven minutes.
  4 . Toward the end, lightly sprinkle tamari over the vegetables, and let the dish sit for several minutes.

  This dish may be eaten up to once a day with a minumum intake of 2 times per week.

- **Azuki, Kombu, and Squash Dish.** To prepare:
  1 . Wash and soak one cup of azuki beans.
  2 . Soak and chop several strips of kombu into one-inch square pieces.
  3 . Place kombu in bottom of pot and add beans.
  4 . Cover with water, bring to a boil, and simmer for 20 minutes.
  5 . Cut hard winter squash (acorn or butternut) into 2-inch chunks, and add kombu and beans.
  6 . Spinkle lightly with sea salt.
  7 . Cover and cook for another 25 to 30 minutes until beans and squash become soft. (If water evaporates, add more from time to time to ensure enough moisture to keep the beans and kombu soft.)
  8 . Add a moderate amount of tamari toward the end of cooking.
  9 . Turn off flame and let vegetables sit for several minutes before serving.

  This dish may be included from 1-3 times per week.

The Importance of Cooking

Macrobiotic cooking is actually very simple once the basic techniques have been mastered. However, before learning the basics, it is very easy to make mistakes, even though various books and publications are consulted. It is very important to attend cooking classes in order to actually see and taste the foods that you wish to prepare. To do this, it isn't necessary to spend a great deal of time attending classes. If you are able to learn at least ten or twenty basic dishes, you can go on to develop your own cooking style. Therefore, when beginning macrobiotics, please seek the advice of friends with experience who live near you. Don't hesitate to show them dishes that you have prepared and ask for their advice and suggestions.

One mistake which is common among cancer patients is the overconsumption of flour products. As much as possible, it is better for a cancer patient to eat grains in their whole form rather than in the form of flour. Flour products easily create mucus and intestinal stagnation, and for this reason it is better to avoid items like cookies, muffins, pancakes, and similar foods. Even high-quality macrobiotic bread should be eaten only several times per week, and not on a daily basis.[15] It is also advisable for cancer patients to avoid heavily baked or grilled foods.

Way of Life Suggestions

1. You may eat regularly, 2-3 times per day provided the proportion is correct and chewing is thorough. Since cancer is a symptom of excess, it is important not to overeat. To prevent this, each mouthful should be thoroughly chewed — at least 100, and preferably 200 times. You may eat as much food as you want provided it is well chewed and thoroughly mixed with saliva, and if you have a tendency to over-eat, be sure to get plenty of physical activity. Therefore, if your strength permits, exercise regularly as a part of daily life, including activities like scrubbing floors, cleaning windows, washing clothes, etc. You may also participate in systematic exercise programs such as yoga, martial arts, or sports.

2. Please avoid eating for three hours before going to bed, as food eaten prior to sleeping will stagnate in the body.

3. Don't watch television for an extended period, directly from the front, or at a close distance, so as to minimize your exposure to radiation. Generally, black and white television transmits a weaker form of radiation than color television.

---

[15]*Flour, diarrhea linked.* "Most people have trouble absorbing all-purpose wheat flour, the kind used to make ordinary white bread, and this may be a previously unsuspected cause of diarrhea and other intestinal problems, a study concludes.

"Researchers found that, when people eat white bread, about 20 percent of it is not absorbed into their digestive tracts. The condition is similar to that experienced by some adults who have difficulty digesting milk.

" 'What it means is that when the average person eats a slice of bread, a fair proportion of it is never absorbed in the small bowel and goes down into the large intestine and can be converted into gas or into stuff that conceivably causes diarrhea,' Dr. Michael D. Levitt, one of the researchers, said.

"The study was conducted at the Veterans Administration Medical Center in Minneapolis and published in today's issue of the *New England Journal of Medicine.*

"Using 18 healthy volunteers, the doctors watched the results when people ate white bread, macaroni, rice bread or bread made from wheat flour that is low in gluten.

"They found that 17 of the 18 persons showed substantial increases in breath hydrogen a few hours after eating six slices of bread." *From the Boston Globe, April 9, 1981.*

4. Try to avoid wearing synthetic or woolen clothing directly on the skin. Use cotton fabrics as much as possible, especially for undergarments and underwear. If, for example, you must wear nylon stockings for social occasions (silk stockings are preferable), remove them as soon as you return. Also, please remove your shoes when you enter your home, so as to allow your feet to breathe and more fully relax. Avoid excessive metallic accessories on the fingers, wrists and neck. Keep such ornaments as simple and graceful as possible.

5. Go outdoors often in simple clothing, barefoot if possible. Try to walk on the grass, soil, or beach for one-half hour whenever the weather permits.

6. Bring many large green plants into your living room or bedroom to freshen and enrich the oxygen content of the air. As much as possible, keep your windows open to allow fresh air to circulate. Don't keep your home too hot in winter, and try to minimize or avoid air conditioning in the summer.

7. Avoid using electric ranges or cooking devices. Convert to gas at the earliest opportunity. Microwave cooking should also be avoided.

8. Use vegetable quality fabrics — especially cotton — for sheets, pillow cases, and blankets.

9. Scrub your entire body with a hot, wet, squeezed towel every morning and every night before sleeping. Place special emphasis on the hands and fingers, feet and toes.

10. Avoid taking long hot baths or showers unless you have been consuming too much salt or animal food.

11. Try to retire before midnight and get up early every morning.

12. Avoid chemically perfumed cosmetics. For care of the teeth, brush with natural preparations or sea salt.

Along with these lifestyle recommendations, we also suggest the following daily reflections:

1. *Develop your appreciation for nature.* Every day, try to set aside several minutes to observe and marvel at the wonder and beauty of our natural surroundings. Appreciate the skies, mountains, sun, wind, rain, snow, and all natural phenomena. Try to regain your sense of marvel at the miracle of life.

2. *View everyone you meet with gratitude, beginning with your family and friends, and extend your gratitude to all people.*

3. *Offer thanks before and after each meal.* Express your gratitude to the sun, earth, air and elements for producing your food, as well as to all those who have grown and prepared it. Use this opportunity to reestablish unity with nature and with society.

The traditional expression, "one grain, ten thousand grains" symbolizes the idea that the earth returns many grains for every one that it receives. A person who is healthy also personifies this ideal in his desire to help others achieve health and happiness.

Therefore, don't hesitate to help other people. Tell them about your experience. As we all know, practically every family is now suffering with cancer, heart disease, or mental illness. If, after you recover, you turn your back on others, it is like hoarding money in a bank account and never using it for your enjoyment. Someone who does this well never become happy, since by helping others, you accelerate your own physical and mental improvement.

When you were born, you never expected to have to sell your time or your life. Exchanging your life for money is not unlike cutting a piece of sausage into slices, weighing it, pricing and offering it to a customer. Please reflect on whether you are really doing what you want to, and try to decide how you want to spend your remaining years of life. If you discover that you are unhappy, begin a process of self-revolution by changing your previous habits and sicknesses into a healthy and sound way of life. With macrobiotics, you can turn your course from one of sickness and decline into one of continuing health and happiness.

Explanation of External Treatments and Natural Applications

1. Ginger Compress

Purpose: Stimulate blood and body fluid circulation; helps loosen and dissolve stagnated toxic matter, cysts, tumors, etc.

Preparation: Place grated ginger in a cheesecloth or cotton sack and squeeze out the ginger juice into a pot of hot water kept just below the boiling point. Dip a towel into the ginger water, wring it out tightly and apply, very hot, directly to the area to be treated. A second, dry towel can be placed on top to reduce heat loss. Apply a fresh hot towel every 2-3 minutes until skin becomes red.

Special Considerations for Cancer Cases: The ginger compress should be prepared in the usual manner. However, it should be applied for only a short time to activate circulation in the affected area, and should be immediately followed by a taro potato plaster. If ginger compress is applied repeatedly over an extended period, it may accelerate the growth of the cancer, particularly if it is a more yin variety. The ginger compress should be considered only as preparation for the taro plaster in cancer cases, not as an independent treatment, and applied for several minutes only. Please seek more specific recommendations from a qualified macrobiotic advisor.

2. Taro Potato (Albi) Plaster

Purpose: Often used after a ginger compress to collect stagnated toxic matter and draw it out of the body.

Preparation: Pare off potato skin and grate the white interior. Mix with 5% grated fresh ginger. Spread this mixture in a ½ inch thick layer onto a piece of fresh cotton linen and apply the taro side directly to the skin. Change every four hours.

Taro potato can usually be obtained in most major cities in the U.S. and Canada, from Chinese, Armenian or Puerto Rican grocery stores or natural foods stores. The skin of this vegetable is brown and covered with "hair." The taro potato is grown in Hawaii as well as in the Orient. Smaller taro potatoes are the most effective for use in this plaster. If taro is not available, a preparation using regular potato can be substituted. While not as effective as taro, it will still produce a beneficial result. Mix 50-60% grated potato with 40-50% grated (crushed) green leafy vegetables, crushing them together in a *suribachi*. Apply as above.

Special Considerations for Cancer Cases: The taro plaster has the effect of drawing cancerous toxins out of the body, and is particularly effective in removing carbon and other minerals which are often contained in tumors. If, when the plaster is removed, the light-colored mixture has become dark or brown, or if the skin where the plaster was applied also takes on a dark color, this change indicates that excessive carbon and other elements are being discharged through the skin. This treatment will gradually reduce the size of the tumor.

If the patient feels chilly from the coolness of the plaster, a hot ginger compress applied for five minutes while changing plasters will help to relieve this. If chill persists, roast sea salt in a skillet, wrap it in a towel, and place it on top of the plaster.

Be careful not to let the patient become too hot from this salt application.

3. Buckwheat Plaster

Purpose: Draws retained water and excess fluid from swollen areas of the body.
Preparation: Mix buckwheat flour with enough hot water to form a hard, stiff dough. Apply in a ½ inch thick layer to the affected area; tie in place with a bandage or piece of cotton linen.
Special Considerations for Cancer Cases: A buckwheat plaster should be applied in cases where a patient develops a swollen abdomen due to retention of fluid. If this fluid is surgically removed, the patient may temporarily feel better, but may suddenly become much worse after several days. It is better to avoid such a drastic procedure.

This plaster can be applied anywhere on the body. In cases where a breast has been removed, for example, the surrounding lymph nodes, the neck, or in some cases the arm, often become swollen after several months. To relieve this condition, apply ginger compresses to the swollen area for about five minutes, then apply a buckwheat plaster; replace every four hours. After removing the plaster, you may notice that fluid is coming out through the skin, or that the swelling is starting to go down. A buckwheat plaster will usually eliminate the swelling after only several applications, or at most after two or three days.

4. Brown Rice Cream: Used to nourish and energize in case of a weakened condition, or when the digestive ability is impaired. Roast brown rice evenly until all the grains turn a yellowish color. To one part rice, add a small amount of sea salt and 3-6 parts water, and pressure cook for at least two hours. Squeeze out the creamy part of the cooked rice gruel with a sanitized cheesecloth. Eat with a small volume of condiment, such as *umeboshi* plum, *gomasio* (sesame salt), *tekka,* kelp or other seaweed powder.

5. Carp Plaster: Reduces high fever, as in the case of pneumonia. Crush and mash a whole, live carp, and mix with a small amount of white wheat flour. Spread this mixture onto an oiled paper and apply to the chest. When treating pneumonia, drink one to two teaspoons of carp blood, and then apply the plaster. Take the body temperature every half hour, and immediately remove the carp plaster when the temperature reaches normal.

6. Daikon Radish Drink: *Drink No. 1:* Will reduce a fever by inducing sweating. Mix half a cup of grated fresh *daikon* with one tablespoon of *tamari* soy sauce and one quarter teaspoon grated ginger. Pour hot *bancha* tea over this mixture, stir and drink while hot. *Drink No. 2:* To induce urination. Use a piece of cheesecloth to squeeze the juice from the grated *daikon.* Mix two tablespoons of this juice with six tablespoons of hot water to which a pinch of sea salt has been added. Boil this mixture and drink only once a day. Do not use this concoction more than three consecutive days without proper supervision and never use it without first boiling.

7. Dentie (Denshi): Prevents tooth problems, promotes a healthy condition in the mouth and stops bleeding anywhere in the body by contracting expanded blood capillaries. Bake an eggplant, particularly the calix or cap, until black. Crush into a powder and mix with 30% to 50% roasted sea salt. Use daily as a tooth powder or apply to any bleeding area — even inside the nostrils in cases of nosebleed — by inserting wet tissue dipped in *dentie* into the nostril.

8. Dried Daikon Leaves: Used to warm to body and to treat various disorders of the skin and female sexual organs. Also helpful in drawing odors and excessive oils from the body. Dry fresh *daikon* leaves in the house, away from direct sunlight, until they turn brown and brittle. (If *daikon* leaves are unavailable, turnip greens can be substituted.) Boil 4-5 bunches of the leaves in 4-5 quarts of water until the water turns brown. Stir in a handful of sea salt and use in one of the following ways:

1. Dip cotton linen into the hot liquid and wring lightly. Apply to the affected area repeatedly, until the skin becomes completely red.
2. Soak in a hot bath in which this mixture has been added.
3. Women experiencing problems in their sexual organs should sit in the bath described above with the water at waist level, the upper portion of the body covered with a towel. Remain in the water until the whole body becomes warm and sweating begins. This generally takes about ten minutes. Repeat as needed, up to ten days.
4. Strain the liquid and use as a douche to eliminate mucus and fat accumulations in the uterine and vaginal regions. This douche can be used after the hot bath described above or by itself.

9. Ginger Sesame Oil: Activates the functions of the blood capillaries, circulation, and nerve reactions. Also relieves aches and pains. Mix grated fresh ginger with an equal amount of sesame oil. Dip cotton linen into this mixture and rub briskly into the skin of the affected area.

10. Grated Daikon: A digestive aid, especially for fatty, oily, heavy foods, and for animal food. Grate fresh *daikon* (red radish or turnip can be used if *daikon* is not available). Sprinkle with *tamari* soy sauce and eat about a tablespoonful.

11. Scallion, Onion, or Daikon Juice: Will neutralize the poison of a bee sting or an insect bite. Cut either a scallion, onion or *daikon,* or their greens, and squeeze out the juice. (If you cannot obtain these vegetables, red radish can be used.) Rub the juice thoroughly into the wound.

12. Kuzu (Kudzu) Drink: Strengthens digestion, increases vitality and relieves general fatigue. Dissolve a heaping teaspoon of *kuzu* powder into one cup of cold water. Bring the mixture to a boil, reduce the heat to the simmering point and stir constantly until the liquid becomes a transparent gelatin. Now stir in one teaspoon of *tamari* soy sauce and drink while hot.

13. Lotus Root Plaster: Draws stagnated mucus from the sinuses, nose, throat and bronchi. Mix grated fresh lotus root with 10%-15% pastry flour and 5% grated fresh ginger. Spread a half-inch layer onto cotton linen and apply the lotus root directly to the skin. Keep on for several hours or overnight, and repeat daily for several days. A ginger compress can be applied before this application to stimulate circulation and to loosen mucus in the area you are treating.

14. Mustard Plaster: Stimulates blood and body fluid circulation and loosens stagnation. Add hot water to dry mustard and stir well. Spread this mixture onto a paper towel, and sandwich it between two thick cotton towels. Apply this "sandwich" until the skin becomes red and warm, and then remove.

15. Ranshio: Used to strengthen the heart, and to stimulate heartbeat and blood circulation. Crush a raw egg and mix with one tablespoon of *tamari* soy sauce. Drink slowly. Use only once a day and for no more than three days.

16. Raw Brown Rice and Seeds: Will eliminate worms of various types. Skip breakfast and lunch. Then, on an empty stomach, eat a handful of raw brown rice with a half-handful of raw seeds such as pumpkin or sunflower seeds, and another half-handful of chopped raw onion, scallion or garlic. Chew everything very well, and have your regular meal later in the day. Repeat for 2 to 3 days.

17. Salt Bancha Tea: Used to loosen stagnation in the nasal cavity or to cleanse the vaginal region. Add enough salt to warm *bancha* tea (body temperature) to make it just a little less salty than sea water. Use the liquid to wash deep inside the nasal cavity through the nostrils, or as a douche. Salt *bancha* tea can also be used as a wash for problems with the eyes.

18. Salt Pack: Used to warm any part of the body. For relief of diarrhea, for example, apply the pack to the abdominal region. Roast salt in a dry pan until hot and then wrap in a thick cotton linen or towel. Apply to the troubled area and change when the pack begins to cool.

19. Salt Water: Cold salt water will contract the skin in the case of burns, while warm salt water can be used to clean the rectum, colon and vagina. When the skin is damaged by fire, immediately soak the burned area in cold salt water until irritation disappears. Then apply vegetable oil to seal the wound from the air. For constipation or mucus and fat accumulations in the rectum, colon, and vaginal regions, use warm salt water (body temperature) as an enema or douche.

20. Sesame Oil: Use to relieve stagnated bowels or to eliminate retained water. Take one to two tablespoons of raw sesame oil on an empty stomach to induce the discharge of stagnated bowels. To eliminate water retention in the eyes, put a drop or two of pure sesame oil in the eyes with an eyedropper, preferably before sleeping. Continue up to a week, until the eyes improve. Before using the sesame oil for this purpose, boil and then strain it with a sanitized cheesecloth to remove impurities.

21. Tamari Bancha Tea: Neutralizes an acidic blood condition, promotes blood circulation and relieves fatigue. Pour one cup of hot *bancha* twig tea over one to two teaspoons of *tamari* soy sauce. Stir and drink hot.

22. Tofu Plaster: Is more effective than an ice pack to draw out a fever. Squeeze the water from the *tofu,* mash it and then add 10%-20% pastry flour and 5% grated ginger. Mix the ingredients and apply directly to the skin. Change every two to three hours.

23. Umeboshi Plum; Baked Umeboshi Plum; Powdered, Baked Umeboshi Plum Pit:
Neutralizes an acidic condition and relieves intestinal problems, including those
caused by microorganisms. Take two or three *umeboshi* plums with *bancha* twig
tea. Or, you may bake the plums or their pits until black. If you are using the pits,
powder them and add a tablespoonful to a little hot water or tea.

24. Ume-Sho-Bancha: Strengthens the blood and the circulation through the regula-
tion of digestion. Pour one cup of *bancha* tea over the meat of one-half to one
umeboshi plum and one teaspoon of *tamari* soy sauce. Stir and drink hot.

25. Ume-Sho-Kuzu (Kudzu) Drink: Strengthens digestion, revitalizes energy and
regulates the intestinal condition. Prepare the *kuzu* drink according to the instructions in Number 12, and add the meat of one-half to one *umeboshi* plum along with
the soy sauce. An eighth of a teaspoon of grated fresh ginger may also be added.

Special Note: *It is generally advisable to use the above special preparations under the
guidance of a qualified macrobiotic advisor.*

CHAPTER TWO
Medical Views

Macrobiotics, Cancer, and Medical Practice

Keith Block, M.D., Penny Block, M.A., Evanston, Illinois

To the modern public, the approach that Dr. Block recommends might sound new and exotic. Actually it is age-old. The staple foods of macrobiotics have been eaten traditionally around the world: brown rice, millet, barley, oats, rye, wheat, corn, and buckwheat. In our practice, the approximate quantities of a basic diet are: 50% cooked whole grains; 25% fresh, local vegetables; 15% beans and sea vegetables; and about 10% fish, soup, condiments, fruits, seeds, and nuts. Of course, it is necessary to modify this food plan for each individual. (see Chapter One.)

People having heard about macrobiotics frequently come with a harvest of questions. The public wants to know, "What foods do I need to eat? Where do I purchase them? How do I prepare them?" Cancer patients and their families — a devoted granddaughter trekking 100 miles to Evanston to gather information; the mother of a 9-year-old cancer victim; the husband of a 29-year-old with a colon malignancy — all are hunting for explanations. At the same time, they are positive in their readiness to pursue a dietary solution to one of modern life's most dread diseases. "What" and "how" are usually ice-breakers before the paramount question surfaces: "Dr. Block, from a medical perspective, why do you think macrobiotics works?"

The marvel is — it does work. And not only for cancer patients. In his practice, Dr. Block has successfully treated people with many afflictions. For John, a strapping 33-year-old suffering from high blood pressure, impotence was the rueful side-effect of his prescribed medication. He was amazed that 6 weeks of macrobiotic eating enabled him to discontinue his drugs comfortably. Up until then, John had resigned himself to a permanent dependence on anti-hypertensives.

It seemed almost miraculous to Jim, a 22-year-old diabetic, that within only three weeks on a macrobiotic regimen, he safely whittled his insulin doses down to less than half of the original prescription. Nighttime shots were called to a halt. For Jim this meant abandoning his former eating style. However, he was so pleased with his rapid improvement that he hardly regretted giving up his old food habits. Even diabetic specialists at the famed Joslin Clinic were blinking their eyes in amazement at the swift results of Jim's diet. Medical professionals at the clinic supported Jim in his eating strategy, after analyzing it carefully. One foresaw that in the coming years all diabetic treatment would rely on a dietary therapy like Jim's.

For 5 years, Jeanine, a woman in her early 40's, had suffered with a urinary tract infection. During this time she had gone to a dozen different G.U. specialists. None of the 17 medications they had prescribed had offered her relief. Not surprisingly, she was growing despondent. When she visited, Dr. Block advised her to stop the medications and begin a basic macrobiotic diet. Due to her specific condition, however, he recommended that she temporarily eliminate fruits, oils, and flour products. One week later, her chronic infection had disappeared; and it didn't reappear. Her words practically skipped along the telephone wire when she called to announce triumphantly, "For the first time in 15 years, I am free of this pesky disorder."

Jeanine's jubilance is representative of many who conscientiously follow their food plans. Relief from illness is not the reward of only a few showcase examples. In the vast experience of Michio Kushi, president of the East West Foundation and author of *The Book of Macrobiotics,* any disorder can find remedy in the macrobiotic diet. From glaucoma to asthma, from herpes to colitis, the results of eating correctly are astonishing.

However, it is cancer which looms as the dread affliction of modern society. One patient confided to Dr. Block that no judge could have delivered a more devastating sentence than the oncologist's words, "terminal cancer." Particularly at night, this patient was haunted by relentless and horrifying images of cancerous growths boring through his body tissue and painfully consuming his life.

Cancer has become epidemic in proportion. According to the American Cancer Society, more than 55 million Americans now living will have cancer in their lifetimes. It will strike 2 out of every 3 families. This could mean that if everyone in your family survives free of cancer, possibly the family living across the hall from you, and another family in the downstairs apartment will lose to cancer. A medical estimate is that by the year 2000, which is only 20 years away, every other person will be stricken with cancer. Of cancer cases, 2/3 are declared incurable. The statistics are staggering and unavoidable. Eleven hundred people per day, one person every 80 seconds is dying in this country of cancer.

Open your newspaper tomorrow and chances are you will read of another household substance, industrial compound, cosmetic ingredient, or even familiar over-the-counter analgesic which has been indicted as a cancer agent. The list of carcinogens now linked with specific occupations, food additives, and environmental contaminants swells with almost unreal speed — like a horror movie monster — at first the size of an ordinary house fly, but suddenly huge enough to overwhelm whole cities.

In *Cancer Care,* written by two M.D.s, Drs. Harold Glucksburg and Jack W. Singer, the modern situation is summarized: "It has been estimated that up to 80% of all cancers are caused or influenced by carcinogens. Until recently, man lived and evolved in a relatively stable and natural environment. This is no longer true. Since the industrial revolution, a dazzling variety of new synthetic products, the effects of which are at best unknown, have been introduced into the environment. We have altered our environment more in the past decade than in the previous millennium."

Like the children's puzzle with pictures that seem intact at first glance but actually conceal several mistakes, such as an upsidedown door or a chimney poking out of the side of a house, our familiar surroundings and daily routines are perforated with cancerous flaws. Publicizing risks has become the daily routine of researchers and media. But bombarded with data, we begin to feel powerless, at times even paranoid.

Then we read of the macrobiotic case histories which indicate the recovery from degenerative disease and discover a possible strategy to overcome cancer. These stories point to hope in a desperate morass of confusion and unknowns.

Again and again, patients call to inquire as to why macrobiotics can heal, and for what reason does the more customary diet hinder health. Although a great deal is yet to be charted scientifically, ample information can be found in medical literature right now. Dr. Block has combed current and old issues of medical periodicals, analyzing data and synthesizing research reports, in order to present the following correlations between food and disorders.

In the foods we eat, additives and preservatives might not be the only culprits that lead to cancer. Some of the familiar staples on the American dinner table have been implicated. Specifically, animal products and refined carbohydrates, which still make up the bulk of the American diet, contain substances which seem to promote disease. Let us review each in more detail.

The Overconsumption of Saturated Fat and Protein

Excessive amounts of saturated fats and cholesterol are abundant in animal foods and dairy products, like beef and butter. Besides the connection between fats and heart/vascular disorders, there is world-wide evidence linking lipids with several forms of cancer. Take colon/rectal cancer for example, one of the most common cancers in the United States. According to a recent study done by Dr. J. P. Cruse and his associates at the University College Hospital Medical School in London, fat consumption has been spotlighted as a cause.

In studying population groups, the highest incidence of colon cancer is witnessed in countries with the highest meat consumption; for example, the United States, Canada, Scotland, and New Zealand. In Japan, where there is less fat intake, bowel cancer occurs less than one-third as frequently as in the U.S. However, if Japanese migrate to the States and adopt a modern, Western diet with its reliance on meat and dairy, they show the same colon cancer statistics as other Americans.

NATIONAL CANCER RATES
(World Health Organization, 1973)

CANCER SITE		DEATH RATE PER 100,000 POPULATION	
		U.S.	Japan
Intestine	Male	17.2	4.6
	Female	19.3	5.0
Breast		29.6	5.4

A fat-laden diet is the chief suspect in other cancers as well. According to the National Cancer Institute, fats accelerate the growth of breast tumors. Hormonal imbalance produced by fats is one explanation given by the American Health Foundation's Dr. Ernst Wynder. In his research he has established that the pancreas, kidney and bladder are also victimized by high fat intake.

In our modern day protein panic, the average person in this country annually consumes 193 pounds of red meat, 53 pounds of poultry, 294 eggs, and 375 pounds of dairy products (including cheese and other milk products.) We've been hooked on a protein-need myth, when actually we might be consuming more than 4 times the protein we require. The present tendency is to assume that "more is better."

The truth is — excessive animal protein intake can jeopardize our health. High protein causes high ammonia levels in the intestines. Dr. Willard Visek, professor of clinical sciences at the University of Illinois Medical School explains: "Ammonia behaves like chemicals that cause cancer or promote its growth. It kills cells ... and it increases the mass of the lining of the intestines. What is intriguing is that within the colon the incidence of cancer parallels the concentration of ammonia."

Even more data exist. In a 1975 issue of the *Journal of Cancer Research,* a high protein diet has been linked to bladder cancer as well as intestinal malignancies. Hesitate before reaching for a second helping and consider this fact. Regardless of the food ingested, excess eating or just plain gorging and gulping can increase tumor size and occurance.

Excessive Dairy Consumption

Many of us have the impression that milk is a pure and wholesome food. However, its fresh, white appearance can be deceiving. Even after processing, milk is still not free of contaminants. An investigation of the Consumers' Union, published in a January 1974 issue of *Consumer Reports,* discovered bacterial counts exceeding 130,000 per milliliter in 7 test samples, although government standards declare safe limits at a maximum of 20,000 bacteria per milliliter (about 1/5 teaspoon.) In fact, one sample contained as much as 3,000,000, and a few contained numbers too large to measure accurately.

In addition, 21 out of 25 tested milk brands were contaminated with pesticides. Health officials concur that there is no level of pesticides in milk that can be judged safe. Also detected in 21 of the milks analyzed were residues of chlorinated hydrocarbons. As they accumulate in the body, these hydrocarbons are not only capable of producing genetic mutations that result in birth defects but also have the potential of forming malignancies.

Added to this is the possibility that the cow milked for the glass you are now filling or for the slice of cheese on your plate might have been infected with bovine C-type virus. In lab experiments, this virus produced leukemia in test animals.

More and more, as explained by Frank Oski, M.D. in his book *Don't Drink Your Milk,* we begin to realize that milk and milk products might not be the benign foods we think they are. Somewhere between 18 months and 4 years, most people begin to lose lactase activity, an enzyme action in the intestines that breaks down lactose, the natural sugar present in milk. Since this decline in lactase is a normal process of maturing, perhaps it was never nature's intention for us to drink milk or eat foods with lactose after the weaning age.

In fact, the vast majority — over two-thirds of people on this earth — are lactose intolerant. So if you continue to drink milk, you might be setting yourself up for a myriad of problems. Some of these include overactivity of mucous secreting glands, infection, and possibly even malignant disease, according to William Crook, who explains the perils of allergenic foods in an article in *Pediatric Clinics of North America.*

Perhaps the most serious indictment of milk and foods derived from milk are the dangers of vitamin D excess and calcification from synthetic vitamin D. In separate medical papers, two M.D.s, Drs. M. Seelig and H. Taussig, have reported the dangerously high, actually toxic levels of vitamin D in our excess consumption of fortified milk products.

In 1953 the problem was aggravated. Major food processors found that it was less expensive to enrich products with an artificial form of the D vitamin, D_2, rather than fortifying with the true from, D_3. In extensive tests conducted by Dr. Hans Selye, a Nobel prize researcher, vitamin D_2 was linked with "Calciphylaxis" or calcium plaquing. There is ample evidence that many diseases, from arteriosclerosis to kidney stones, can be traced to this deleterious process of calcification. Microscopic- examinations of cancer tumors frequently reveal calcium deposits. Why this link between tumors and calcification occurs, science has not yet documented. But the fact remains, the connection does exist.

Refined Carbohydrates and Sugar

Refined carbohydrates and processed foods have been judged guilty of many modern day woes. One of the most obvious is tooth decay. But the hazards of sugar are considerable. It plays an active role in such disorders as hyperactivity and diabetes, and creates a susceptibility to polio, other infectious diseases, ulcers, and heart disease. Add to this catalogue of incriminations — cancer.

In a study commissioned by Hoffman-La Roche, Inc., sucrose (sugar) and xylitol (a substance used to sweeten sugarless gum) were found to produce malignant liver tumors. Although the test results were released in March 1978, the FDA did not discuss them with the Federal Trade Commission until the following year. Many researchers believe that if sugar were first introduced today, it would stand little chance of being approved by the FDA for mass consumption. Due to these lab tests, xylitol is not used commonly today, while sugar is still ever-present. In fact, it's almost impossible to wander through the grocery aisles and locate a can or package that does not include sugar in its contents. Moreover, sugar can be cleverly concealed on labels behind an alias like "sucrose" or "dextrose."

Solution: 1 — Whole Cereal Grains

In travelling from farm field to grocery shelf, processed and packaged grain products have been stripped of most vitamins and minerals. Robbed of nature's rich nutrients, these refined carbohydrates are then stuffed with artificial supplements. In contrast, whole grains are "the real thing."

Professor Paul C. Mangelsdorf in the July 1963 issue of *Scientific American* made this definitive statement: "Cereal grains ... represent a five-in-one food supply which contains carbohydrates, proteins, fats, minerals, and vitamins. A whole grain cereal, if its food values are not destroyed by the over-refinement of modern processing methods, comes closer than any other plant product to providing an adequate diet."

Whole grains heal the body as well as fuel it. High fiber, the stuff of cereal grains, reduces the risk of colon and other cancers. As an additional bonus, grains produce a beneficial form of cholesterol. Unlike the harmful type associated with animal foods, this favorable cholesterol actually breaks down dangerous saturated fat and oil residue.

Perhaps most impressive is the role grains can play in strengthening the entire immunologic system, the body's equipment in combatting disease. A May 1980 issue of *Hospital Tribune* reports that diseases stemming from a weak immune system "are associated with a high incidence of malignancies."

Three vitamins in particular are essential to immunity: pyridoxine (vitamin B_6),

45

folic acid, and pantothenic acid. All are plentiful in whole grains. According to Dr. A. E. Axelrod of Pittsburgh University Medical School, if any one of these three is absent from the diet, the body cannot manufacture antibodies (proteins that fight disease.) Unfortunately, it is these three elements of the B-complex that are left on the milling room floor in the refining process. Therefore, they are not present in white bread, white flour products, white rice, or even degerminated cornmeal. The implications of this are tremendous: A natural, whole grain diet can build resistance to disease, while a refined foods diet does not.

Solution: 2 — Miso

Said Philippe Shubik in *Potential Carcinogenicity of Food Additives and Contaminants,* "Since it might not be possible to remove all carcinogenic materials from the environment, methods to mitigate or neutralize their harmful effects should be sought." Surprisingly, the sought-after substance might not emerge from chemical labs and test-tube concoctions but from less obvious sources: fermented soybeans and sea vegetables.

Miso (pronounced mee-so), a deep and rich tasting fermented soybean purée, appears regularly in macrobiotic menus, especially soups and condiments. An excellent provider of protein, B_{12} and other nutrients, it boasts properties that work almost like magic in the body. When the atomic bomb was dropped on Nagasaki in 1945 , Dr. Akizuki, director of Urakame Hospital, made certain that his entire staff was fed miso soup daily. Exposure to radiation was unavoidable; his hospital was located only one mile form the center of the blast. In follow-up studies, he discovered that none of his co-workers suffered from the devastating effects of atomic radiation. Other comparable groups were not as fortunate. He hypothesized that miso was the protective factor.

Almost 30 years later, in 1972, Japanese scientists who were stimulated by Dr. Akizuki's records identified *Zybicolin* in miso. This substance, a byproduct of the natto and miso yeasts, has been found to collect and then remove from the body heavy molecules — metals, pollutants, and radioactive poisons.

Miso has a repertoire of other benefits. For one, it is richly endowed with lecithin and linoleic acid. Each of these dissolves, then eliminates cancer-linked cholesterol and fat accumulations. Another benefit: An acid blood condition is like a door thrust open to disease. Miso helps to shut this door by modulating an acid blood level into a healthy alkaline level. And an additional bonus: Present in all non-pasteurized misos are active enzymes, particularly *lactobacillus,* which aid the digestive flora.

Solution: 3 — Sea-Vegetables

If someone mentions treasures from the sea, we usually picture pirate chests bursting with gold pieces. Actually, simple plants growing in the ocean yield rich bounties for our health and well-being.

Put aside your vitamin capsules and mineral supplements. Sea grown vegetables furnish copious amounts of vitamins A, B, and C. One variety *kombu,* a popular macrobiotic soup ingredient, has three times more B vitamins than milk or milk products. And Ergosterol, which converts to vitamin D (the natural version, D_3) in the body, is richly supplied by all sea plants.

In addition, mineral assets are high in sea vegetables. For example, an average portion of *hiziki* provides 14 times the quantity of calcium found in a glass of milk. No other food source can claim as great a concentration of iron as *dulse*. Another boon: Research has found that cancer sufferers excrete vital amounts of zinc; kelp readily replenishes this essential element.

Besides this rich inventory of vitamins, minerals and basic nutrients, sea vegetables, actually inhibit the absorption of radioactive strontium and cadmium. Further, in research at McGill University, Montreal, alginates demonstrated the ability to bind with heavy, toxic molecules within the intestines and then to change them into insoluble salts which are finally excreted from the body.

Unlike prescription medications, whole grains, miso and sea vegetables do not produce the harmful side effects often connected with drugs. Macrobiotics is, therefore, not only good food. It is also good medicine.

It is sad truth that in the declared "war against cancer" no new drug treatment nor modern medical technology has produced any true victories. According to Dr. Robert Mendelsohn, author of *Confessions of a Medical Heretic* and former chairman of the Medical Licensing Board of the State of Illinois, "In the closing decades of the 20th century, the great scourges of our time are heart disease and cancer; both are regarded as mysterious and despite (or because of?) all the efforts of modern medicine, still incurable." Thus, macrobiotics is not only good medicine, it might be one of the few effective ones.

However, some patients discover that switching from American staples to a macrobiotic diet might not be a simple one-step procedure. For many people, changing the foods they eat means changing their lives. Realigning personal priorities is involved. Each of us must weigh the importance of our health against the comfort of our habits.

Perhaps cancer will not become an obsolete term in this, or even the next generation. But shrugging our shoulders in despair and surrendering to disease are not necessary. Even though we cannot immmediately purge all the carcinogens from our external environment, we can, as promptly as our next meal, begin to clean house internally.

New Directions in Modern Medicine

Robert S. Mendelsohn, M.D., Chicago, Illinois

The following article is from an address
at the Foundation's 1980 Cancer Conference.

I would like to review several of the more positive changes that have taken place in modern medicine since I met with you at last year's conference. I would also like to offer a number of predictions about the future.

I am aware of at least eight advances in medicine over the last year:

1. Three months ago, the American Medical Association came out against the routine annual physical exam. I consider this to be a major breakthrough. The annual physical exam has been, until now, one of the major rituals in modern medicine. It has existed since the Great Depression when doctors did not have enough business, so they decided that everyone should have an exam every year. They were quickly followed by dentists, and both groups rapidly turned to x-rays.

    The routine physical exam has become so counterproductive that the AMA has to come out against it. When I heard this, I thought that they must have read my book, *Confessions of a Medical Heretic,* because the chapter that deals with the annual physical exam is entitled, "If This Is Preventive Medicine, I'll Take My Chances with Disease." My prediction is that now that the routine annual physical exam (and their x-rays) is being proscribed, the incidence of cancer will certainly drop. So I am very happy to see the AMA come out against the routine physical exam.

2. Two months ago, the American Cancer Society came out against the routine annual chest x-ray. Now when I saw that happen, I could hardly believe it. I could not believe that modern medicine could move so fast in one year. I think it is quite clear that x-rays play a part in the causation of cancer. We know that mammography, used to detect breast cancer, can certainly cause breast cancer, and I do not think there is any question that now that we are getting rid of the annual examination of the chest by x-ray, the incidence of cancer is going to go down.

3. Two and a half months ago, the American Cancer Society came out against the routine annual Pap smear, and that interested me because the incidence of error in the Pap smear is somewhere between 20% and 30%. Also, there is no evidence, throughout the two decades that the Pap smear has been in existence, of any change in the mortality or incidence of cervical cancer between areas where the Pap smear is extensively used and areas where it is not used at all. Since the error rate is so high, my prediction is that the dropping of the routine annual Pap smear will also result in a drop in the rate of cancer.

4. This year, sales of Valium dropped by 30%. Now I do not want to take the credit for that, even though I am willing to take the credit; because I always take credit for things I do not deserve to make up for the blame for things I do not deserve. But in this case, I have to give credit to a woman who wrote a book called *I'm Dancing As Fast As I Can.* Her name is Barbara Gordon.

The book tells how to get off of Valium, which doctors don't know how to tell you. Doctors tell you how to get on drugs. But they do not tell you how to get off.

5. The national tripling of home births is my next area of praise. This has surprised me because I never thought that so many people would opt out of the temple of modern medicine and decide to carry out the sacrament of birth at home instead of in a hospital. Because, as you know, modern medicine likes you to carry out the sacrament of birth and the sacrament of death inside the temple; in both cases this works at destroying your family. Recently obstetricians will allow you to have your husband with you, but they still snatch away the baby and put him or her into a newborn nursery.

    At the other end of life, of course, you have to die under conditions of intensive care where the visiting hours are five minutes out of every hour, and you have 55 minutes to die with no family or friends around; where there is only a monitor to hear your last words. (I come from a generation where the word "monitor" meant "hallguard," and I still have trouble with that word.)

6. The next advance is the recently announced recommendation of the National Institutes of Health, which is only a few weeks old, against automatic repeat Caeserian sections and against automatic sections for breech babies. Now that surprised me because as most of you know, the incidence of sections has risen from a normal rate of 4% or 5% to somewhere between 20% and 40%. And in large research and teaching hospitals, some of which are here in Boston, the rates have been found to be over 50%. That is due to the mistaken notion that "once a section always a section." I thought it would take over 20 years before we could get rid of what I call "the old doctor's tale." And here it disappears just a few months ago. One week ago, I debated on television with George Ryan, M.D., who is the incoming president of the American College of Obstetrics and Gynecology. He said on television that doctors were already giving up automatic repeat sections and automatic sections for breech babies. (One of the cardinal beliefs of modern medicine is that God made a mistake when he did not put a zipper in every woman's belly.) Obstetricians in general believe that the best way to have a baby is by Caesarian section, but they do not say exactly that. They turn to religious terms. As an example, they often say "Would you not rather have your baby from above than below?" And since the expression "from above" has the aura of divinity about it, who wants to have a baby from below?

7. The next advance is the action of my own organization, the American Academy of Pediatrics, endorsing breastfeeding; only 23 years behind the La Leche League. This action also violates one of the beliefs of modern medicine, since pediatricians have always felt that God made a mistake when He did not put Similac in women's breasts. But now they are endorsing breastfeeding and the incidence has risen in this country from 15% in the 1960's to a present rate of 63%. I predict that soon infant formula will finally be recognized as the "granddaddy of all junk food."

8. The next advance is the recently announced Food and Drug Administration action to remove three thousand drugs from the market. I do not know how many of you saw that in you paper. It was in the *Washington Post*.

These are the eight major advances in modern medicine over the past year which I think will mark at turnaround. Now all of modern medicine is beginning to backpedal as quickly as it possibly can. It is even beginning to take credit for the drop in cancer incidence and mortality that I predict will happen. And I am perfectly happy to give them credit. For as far a I can tell, as soon as doctors stop practicing the kind of medicine they have been practicing over the last 40 years, the incidence of cancer is bound to go down.

Now I want to give you some idea what has happened inside of medicine, because some of you might not have had the opportunity to keep up with all the recent medical journals. One of the studies that I have been quoting for a long time is twelve years old. It comes from a book by two British doctors, named, appropriately enough, Sharp and Keene. The name of the book is *Presymptomatic Detection and Early Diagnosis*. This study, done in England, showed that the Pap smear was valueless, and that there was no difference in the incidence or mortality in those who used the Pap smear and those who did not.

The same study was repeated last year by two doctors from New York University and Yale. The doctor from New York is Dr. Annemarie Foltz, and the one from Yale is Jennifer L. Kelsey. They pointed out that it has not been well established that the screening of large numbers of women has had any effect on the death rate from cervical cancer. Questioning the current medical practice of the yearly Pap smear on adult women, these researchers state that there is a 20-30% incidence of false negatives found, to say nothing of the incidence of false positives. They point out the questionable accuracy in the test, and also the fact that it became standard recommended policy without ever having been subjected to controlled trials to determine its efficacy.

The next item is from Francis Straus, Professor of Pathology, at my own University of Chicago. Dr. Straus pointed out the technical problem associated with biopsies. I want to quote several sentences which describe things that can go wrong. This is from a publication *Cancer News for Physicians,* published in the fall of 1979. As Dr. Straus points out, once the biopsy sample has been delicately removed from the patient, it is not out of danger. It is all too easy to lay the biopsy down on a sterile prep tray, (if you have ever stood in an operating room, you might know exactly how true this is), or to become engrossed in repairing a surgical defect while the tiny morsel desicates into a tiny unrecoverable shadow of its former self, compressed by distortion from repeated picking up by forceps' teeth or squeezing through fingertips. I cannot tell you how often I have seen this, especially in research and teaching hospitals where everybody has to squeeze that biopsy to feel if it is soft or hard. (This also happens to women in labor, as everyone has to come in and do a vaginal exam — intern, resident doctor, nurse, cleaning lady, etc.)

Straus continues to caution us — i.e., one important but often overlooked aspect of performing a biopsy is the cleanliness and sharpness of the biopsy instrument. Frequently the biopsy tool contains tissue fragments from the previous biopsy which dry and later are autoclaved with the instrument. Such desicated particles impair the function of the instrument and confuse the pathologist (all we need is a confused pathologist) when mixed with the current specimen. Many cup forceps biopsies are torn off, because the cutting edge of the instrument has been allowed to become blunted through continual use.

Here is an item from John Gofman, M.D., Ph.D., and an expert on leukemia.

Dr. Gofman points out that each year dental and medical diagnostic x-rays are responsible for 12,000 extra fatal cancers. He also points out that when the technician takes the x-ray, as many as one extra film per three is common — only taken to correct for errors. And for those of you who are interested in sexism and medicine, watch who goes in to take the x-rays and then watch who reads the x-rays. In my experience, it is almost always the male doctors who sit in their office and read the x-rays, while the female technician actually takes them.

Arthur Upton, director of the National Cancer Institute, pointed out the risk of x-rays to radiologists, including a strong association with leukemia, skin cancer, lymphoma, and cancer of the brain. I always knew that radiologists had a higher incidence of leukemia, but I did not know they also had these other diseases. X-ray treatment for arthritis of the spine can produce an increased risk of cancer of the pancreas, leukemia, and other neoplasms. As the same time, studies on pregnant women have revealed that prenatal exposure to x-rays involving a dose on the order of one rad (that is what you get from one chest x-ray or from a full-mouth dental x-ray) are associated with a 50% increase in the risk of childhood leukemia. According to the *British Medical Journal,* children born to hospital anesthetists are sixty times more likely to suffer from cancer than other children. The incidence of breast cancer in women anesthetists was also found to be fifty times higher than normal Exposure to anesthetics can cause problems ranging from cleft lips and cleft palates to severe neurologic difficulties, bone and muscle disorders, impaired intellectual development, a low birth rate, and a higher incidence of miscarriage among anesthetists. Thirty percent of the anesthetists studied had problems getting pregnant.

Every once in a while a treatment for cancer comes out that is claimed to be perfectly safe. I am used to that, because one of the rules in medicine is to always use a new drug as quickly a you can before the side effects become known. So, for example, these days, ultra-sound, amniocentecis and bilirubin lights are being extensively used, even though we already know the dangers of those procedures. Vasectomy is another procedure which is still used extensively (over a million operations a year) even though the dangers of vasectomy are already known.

As far as cancer is concerned, a new drug came out a few years ago called Tamoxifen, which is used in certain cases of cancer of the breast. Here is the latest description of its side effects. This drug might produce oncogenic activity in animals. For those of you who do not know Greek, oncogenic means tumor-producing. I am very interested in chemotherapeutic agents causing cancer, because Interferon, which I am sure you are going to hear more about, comes in four types. One type, Lymphoblastoid Interferon, can cause cancer according to the press release sent out by Searle Laboratories. I did not see one newspaper pick that up. So now if your doctor wants to give you Interferon, ask him which kind.

Now here is an item from *Lancet,* March 15, 1980. This prestigious medical journal reports that the overall survival rate of patients with primary breast cancer has not improved in the last 10 years despite increasing use of multiple drug chemotherapy for treatment of metastases. Furthermore, there has been no improvement in survival from the first metastasis, and survival might have even been shortened in some patients given chemotherapy.

Many patients come to me because they want to know whether or not they should go for chemotherapy. My answer is always to ask you doctor whether he has any study on patients who have refused chemotherapy. The doctor will probably tell you they have no studies because they do not follow up on those patients. However, he will probably tell you that they have an 80% cure rate on those they do follow up on. My answer to that is "how do you know that the other group does not have a 90% cure rate?" But if you want to, you can always take up the *Lancet* article with your doctor, although I warn you to be careful, because your doctor might fire you. This is one of those strange financial interactions in life where the employee can fire the employer. If he does not actually dismiss you as a patient, the doctor might get angry with you, because there are only two things that doctors do not like to hear from patients. I owe this line to David Stewart, Ph.D., who is head of NAPSAC (National Association of Parents and Professionals for Safe Alternatives in Child-birth), who says that the only things doctors do not like to hear are: (1) something they already know, and (2) something they do not know. Otherwise, they are always ready to listen to anything as long as it does not take too long.

I am now going to go on to my predictions. My first prediction is that more and more people are going to be turning to alternative systems. I cannot tell you strongly enough how grateful I am to meet with all of you and to thank you for introducing me to macrobiotics as something I can offer my patients. The macrobiotic move-ment, which once was regarded as out of the mainstream, has now become very mainstream as a result of the activities of the Senate Nutrition Committee, as well as meetings such as those held by Michio Kushi and the East West Foundation in Washington.

Macrobiotics, and other similar nutritional approaches, are going to gain increas-ingly large audiences. However, macrobiotics in particular has several distinct ad-vantages which guarantee it an ever-ascending place in American society. I predict that we are going to gather here in several years, and the AMA is going to say that the reason why the rate of cancer has diminished is because of their activities such as those mentioned earlier in this presentation. We are going to claim that the cancer rate went down because the nutritional habits of the people have changed. Both sides are right.

In conclusion, let me present three ways in which macrobiotics is different from conventional nutritional science:

Number 1: Macrobiotics appreciates and emphasizes the crucial importance of societal, cultural and familial background in determining proper dietary patterns. I think that this is crucial in understanding that diet is only part of the whole.

Number 2: Macrobiotics appreciates and emphasizes the crucial importance of pre-natal nutrition and breastfeeding in determining the future development of each indi-vidual. I think that this is very important because the other systems that I have looked at do not emphasize strongly enough the effect of prenatal and infant nutrition.

Number 3: Macrobiotics appreciates and emphasizes the crucial importance of incorporating diet into a universal system of thought and behavior. It does not get caught in the trap of singling out cholesterol or vitamins or trace minerals or pro-tein. Macrobiotics is a synthesizing system. American nutrition in contrast depends on analysis. Some of you who are interested in psychiatry might remember one of the rules of psychiatry which states that after your patient has spent enough time in analysis, he develops a state of inaction known as "paralysis through analysis."

My final prediction is that cancer will eventually be conquered, not through surgery, x-ray treatments or chemotherapy — not even by laetrile. Cancer will be conquered by the profound wisdom of leaders like Michio Kushi and universal truths like macrobiotics.

Tomorrow, here in Boston, I will be appearing on a number of television and radio shows, as I am in the middle of a thirty-city book tour. I plan to make sure that everyone who interviews me knows that the reason I am here is to attend this Conference and to learn from the East West Foundation about macrobiotics and everything that it stands for. I know that all of you will carry this important message back to your own communities and I can tell you that those of us in Chicago who belong to the Foundation's Medical/Scientific Advisory Committee are certainly going to do our best. I would like you to know that I think your attendance here today is evidence not only of the value of macrobiotics in your own personal lives, but evidence of the continuous advance of macrobiotics on the American scene.

Thank you very much.

Macrobiotics and Mutual Support

Peter Klein, M.D., Washington, D. C.

The following article is from an address at the Foundation's 1980 Cancer Conference. It includes an account of Dr. Klein's use of macrobiotics in his recovery from hyperlipidemia and related problems.

It was four years ago that I first heard about macrobiotics, after attending an introductory talk in Los Angeles. Following the lecture, most of us sat down to a macrobiotically prepared meal which began with miso soup and included grains and vegetables. I enjoyed the food and the company of the people I met. As I chewed my food, I began to think that this was something I should have started long ago. The meals got better and better as my sensitivity to taste improved, and I soon realized that I was doing something that could lead to a change in my health and well being.

The idea of improving my health through natural methods had been evolving in me for quite a while, but the pressure and pace of my work and education, and especially of medical school, had left less and less time. However, in some ways I had come close to the macrobiotic diet. Once I had found it, though, I realized I was beginning a study that would involve unlearning as well as learning.

Eating macrobiotically has done a lot for me. It helped bring my cholesterol level down to normal and I now feel that the quality of my blood will continue to improve, along with the condition of my blood vessels and my condition in general. I no longer worry about the degeneration of blood vessels that plagued me when I found out that I had type IV hyperlipidemia.

The macrobiotic diet also helped lower my blood sugar level to normal; thus I stopped worrying about diabetes with its degeneration of the small arteries, "blindness," impotency, strokes, heart attacks, amputations, and nerve losses. Macrobiotics has also helped me with the fears of gout, with its associated arthritis, possible kidney stones, and renal problems.

Since beginning to eat macrobioticaly, I have had fewer colds, upper respiratory and throat infections, stomach upsets, and similar chronic problems, plus fewer conscious and unconscious fears about illness in general. This has been a great relief to me, since I have been plagued with illness from childhood, starting with an early reaction to cow's milk and the development of allergies, to severe asthma at the age of three. From then on I had difficulty in breathing and frequently stayed up all night until I discovered that if I rocked back and forth in bed, I would eventually pass out. However, I never knew if I would wake up or suffocate, and when I did wake up, I knew there would be another night of struggle.

After three episodes of severe upper respiratory infection, the last being a case of pneumonia, I was hospitalized and placed in an oxygen tent for several months. After this, I went to an asthmatic home in Denver. For the first time in life, I was free to play football, baseball, basketball, etc., and my condition improved. However, when I returned home, I occasionally had an attack until I moved to New Orleans to go to medical school.

While I was in medical school, my mother's doctor discovered that she had type IV hyperlipidemia and started her on Atronoid S. As soon as I found this out, I ran a test which showed that I also had type IV hyperlipidemia, along with a uric acid of 13.5 (normal is about 6). Hyperuricemia is usually a precursor of gout, and my elevated blood sugar (10) a possible precursor of diabetes. Afterwards, my brother was tested and found to have a uric acid count of about 11. He decided to go on drug therapy. I decided I was not going to take any drugs, especially the one recommended for me, since I knew one out of a thousand people who took it developed leukemia, which is what my father had died from. I concluded that I must be putting something into my body that was causing me to have an abnormal chemistry, and decided to figure out how to get myself back in balance.

I decided to start by giving up animal foods, because their high protein content is converted to purine, which eventually shows up as uric acid. Animal foods such as dairy products and eggs are also high in the things that elevate the lipid level. I also started to eliminate sugar and sweets, since they often compromise the pancreas.

I had a lot to learn and, as a medical student, not much time to do it, especially since I had to work as many as 39 hours a week to pay my way through medical school. However, even though I had some idea of the foods I had to give up, I did not know what to eat and how to prepare it. The medical literature on nutrition was of little help, since I could not find diets that excluded animal food and sugar, while the recommended substitutes were usually highly processed or synthetic foods.

During medical school I began to see more and more how the intake of certain substances contributed to illness and degeneration. It was easy to see how alcohol contributed to liver disease, pancreatitis and gastrointestinal problems, and how diets high in animal foods, dairy and eggs contributed to cardiovascular disease, as did obesity in general. It was also obvious that sugar could lead to the development of hypoglycemia and mild maturity onset diabetes, with related cardiovascular problems, heart attacks, strokes, blindness, impotency and amputations. I also saw how smoking and air pollution led to lung disease, and from my personal experience realized how milk and orange juice led to mucus deposits which contributed to difficulty in breathing and asthma. I also saw how stress and the rapid pace of life led to tension and possible hypertension, and how quick decisions based on poor judgement led to frequent accidents and mistakes.

As I became more observant of human behavior, it became obvious that many people had fixed patterns of thinking that prevented them from searching deeper and figuring out better and more enjoyable ways of doing things. During my internship in Los Angeles, I came to the conclusion that it would be much better to do whatever was necessary to prevent illness than to try and treat it once it developed. From working with many sick people, I saw how difficult it was to try to help them once their sickness had become acute. I had never worked so hard and seen so much tragedy, pain and frustration.

At some point I realized that hospitals and medicine were not going to provide the knowledge I was seeking, since they were concerned mostly with treating disease. After completing my internship, I started my psychiatry residency and took a job working at an emergency room on weekends. It was there that I treated an architect who introduced me to the East West Center in Los Angeles.

It was here that my exploration of macrobiotics began. It has been interesting, exciting, unique, perplexing and at times difficult, but I have continued to learn and my health has continued to improve. I have occasionally had reactions when I have decided to eat or try something that is not right for me. Whether I am aware of it or not, this disturbs the balance I am establishing, and thus I always learn from these experiences, eventually making the appropriate adjustments.

With that in mind I began to study individual and family development. I have frequently found that those who function best come from families that are physically, emotionally, intellectually and socially supportive, while appropriately setting beneficial limits that are not restrictive.

In order to help people make positive changes in their way of life, they need the same kind of support, encouragement and nurturance that a family and friends provide. I therefore use group therapy to help patients, with the group becoming a new pseudo-family which fosters beneficial development by providing an opportunity to share ideas on how to improve one's interactions with oneself, with others, and with the environment.

I would like to emphasize that you too can benefit from the support and encouragement of others who share your interest and desire for better health. Regular contact with them can facilitate emotional, intellectual and social well being, along with physical improvement. Group activities such as dinners, discussions, group walks, exercises and others offer pleasant and enjoyable opportunities to share what you have done that has helped you. I would like to advise you to introduce yourselves to other macrobiotic people and exchange information with them on a regular basis.

For me, it is very enriching and rewarding to be involved in sharing with and helping others. My work is with the illnesses of greed, arrogance and disharmony that we have created and spread in this world. I would like to ask you to do what you can both for yourself and for others who need and will appreciate your help. It is from here that the proper understanding of how to create health will continue to spread to all who need and want it.

New Dimensions in Nursing

Kristen Schmidt, R.N., Allston, Massachusetts

*Kristen Schmidt, a registered nurse, is currently studying
at the Kushi Institute in Brookline, Massachusetts,
and is active in the Macrobiotic Nurses Guild in Boston.*

It is common knowledge that there is an upheaval in nursing today. In February of this year, the American Hospital Association held a national investigation which revealed that nurses are leaving the profession because of economic, political, educational, and status deficits. However, I would like to suggest that the underlying reason is much deeper; nurses have lost their dream. To me, a dream has something to do with aesthetics and intangibles; not so much with material acquisitions or prestige. I'll share with you my own dream upon entering nursing school, and in so doing reflect on what other nurses' aspirations are as well.

I had hoped to achieve a sense of personal growth, worth, and actualization. I wanted to have intimate contact with people and effect a change in their lives. I wanted to contribute something valuable to society, and to strengthen and work with people's support system. In becoming a nurse, I hoped to be able to directly influence a person's health. Working with the patient and family would be working with a mini-society. But most exciting and challenging was the idea that there is a creative art to the profession of care for people.

The Traditional Nurse

Nursing has always been in existence; it is not necessary to go to school to become a nurse. In America, the profession of nursing began when the Civil War demanded the need for an organization of women to care for the sick and wounded. After the war, "centers of hospitality" arose, but often the nurse went to the home. In the course of aiding in patient's recovery, the nurse had a wide range of responsibilities. She provided personal care by bathing, grooming, massaging and exercising the patient. Medically, the nurse prepared and administered herbal medications, applied external plasters, fomentations and compresses. She was an acute observer of her patient's emotions, behavior, and response to physical stimuli. In care of the patient's surroundings, she brightened or darkened the "sick room" depending upon his or her need. The room was kept clean and orderly. A soothing emotional environment was provided to induce relaxation which enhanced the healing process. Part of her day was spent reading and conversing with her patient.

The nurse was a liaison between the patient and family. Information was gathered from the family to aid in her assessment and plan of care. Frequent reports of the patient's changing condition were mediated by the nurse. Since she was closest to the patient during his illness, she did collaborative work with the physician. He depended on her observations and intuition to make his diagnosis and formulate a treatment plan.

Education of the patient and family was another responsibility. In simple terms, she explained how to restore and maintain health.

Perhaps the nurse's most sagacious and powerful role was that of moral counselor. She understood that along with sickness comes regression, depression, and dependency. Having nothing to do and nowhere to go, the patient would often re-examine the priorities in his life. Her counsel and assistance for the patient's self-reflection were always available. The old schools of nursing taught that the nurse should be cheerful and optimistic. She was the patient's biggest advocate. Her intention for a good recovery set the tone for everything she did with her patient. She was an inspiration to his confidence, providing constant encouragement and support. Above all, she understood that personality and behavior were not independent of scientific knowledge and medicine.

Traditional and Macrobiotic Nursing

What the nurse used to do made her function valuable and gave her a sense of autonomy because she saw a direct improvement from her interactions with the patient. She was realizing her dream. Nurses today spend more time interacting with machines than patients; as a result, they are not directly responsible for positive results. Their self worth is challenged.

The traditional nurse and macrobiotic nurse are consorts. They both show an awareness as to whether a patient's overall energy is functioning properly. During the course of daily patient care this can be accomplished in various ways:

1. Touch

Energy runs through twelve pathways (meridians) in the body. Touch subtly but powerfully affects the quality of energy flowing through the meridians.[1] The traditional nurse was well educated in the technique and importance of massage, bathing, external applications and general personal care of her patient. Her touch was an art, highly regarded by the patient. Macrobiotics teaches *Shiatsu* (pressure point massage) and acupuncture. Both are used to stimulate and release energy, as diagnostic tools, as methods of analgesia and anesthesia, and in the treatment of illness.

2. Nutrition

The old school recognized the importance of high quality, well balanced and properly cooked food, both as a vehicle to recovery and as an intergral part of the maintenance of good health. Macrobiotics teaches that foods such as whole grains, beans, and vegetables, which were the traditional foods of our ancestors, provide the optimum balance of all the necessary nutrients to enhance a healthy body, keeping the mind and body clear for the free flow of energy.

3. Emotional Interaction

The traditional and macrobiotic nurse both help the patient express his concerns and feelings. Talking, crying, laughing, and singing are extractions of emotional energy. Verbal interchange transfers energy between the patient and nurse. Often, the patient will feel relaxed and relieved after a good conversation. Compassion and the intent of wellness are in a sense high quality "emotional food" offered by the nurse to her patient.

---

[1] Please refer to the *Book of Do-In: Exercise for Physical and Spiritual Development* by Michio Kushi (Japan Publications) for a discussion of the energy meridians which have been used for thousands of years in the practice of acupuncture, Shiatsu, Do-In (self-massage) and other traditional Oriental therapies.

4. Observation

Before the advent of machinery as a tool for charting and observation, the nurse of yesteryear relied on her six senses (sight, sound, touch, hearing, taste, perception) as tools for monitoring her patient's changing condition. This was a well developed art and science. Observations of body flexibility and tension, pain threshhold, skin color, texture, and temperature, bodily smell, the patient's voice and body sounds (i.e., bowel peristalisis, rales in lungs), and behavioral patterns were all important factors in this process. She had an understanding that the external manifestation of signs and symptoms reflected the internal condition of the body.

The macrobiotic methods of diagnosis are easily integrated in this process.[2] Certain areas of the face and body relate directly to organs and systems (digestive, reproductive, respiratory, circulatory, nervous, endocrine). With these methods, a nurse can immediately understand the patient's condition before the manifestation of physical signs and symptoms. This method can be valuable because it does not have the danger of side effects, nor the expense of extensive technological testing.

Studies

What are some of the tangible effects of these methods in the restoration of a patient's health today?

1. Touch

Delores Krieger, R.N., Ph.D. (Professor of Nursing, New York University) began her practice and research into therapeutic touch in 1969. She theorizes that there is a transfer of energy from healer to patient that is "done physiologically by a kind of electron transfer resonance" (1). At the Langly Porter Neuropsychiatric Institute, U.C.L.A., San Francisco, her methodology was tested with highly sophisticated equipment. "Mr. A. ... had had severe neck and back pain for several years following the injection of contrast dye into the spinal canal for myographic studies. Since then, he had been unable to walk down a flight of stairs without the aid of crutches." After therapeutic touch, "Mr. A. walked out of the laboratory, down a standard flight of stairs, and out to the street carrying his crutches ... " (2) A woman with fibroid tumors, upon follow-up examination after therapeutic touch, had no tumors to be found in her uterus. In another case, the severity of chronic migraine headaches in a young woman was diminished.

Ms. Krieger's technique is being taught as a part of the Master's Program in nursing at New York University and is presented in universities and hospitals throughout the United States. Other nurses have followed Ms. Krieger's path and found this method of vibrational healing to be beneficial in the patients they treat (3).

2. Nutrition

Michio Kushi has found that the quality of food can be directly responsible for the cause, and in many instances, the relief of most degenerative diseases. Whole grains, vegetables, beans, and other natural, traditional foods contain the highest quality nutritional energy. When cooked properly and eaten on a daily basis, more balanced foods can heal the body naturally and completely. The case histories in this volume offer examples of this.

---

[2]Please refer to *How to See Your Health: The Book of Oriental Diagnosis* by Michio Kushi (Japan Publications) for a discussion of these traditional methods.

3. Emotion

Norman Cousins' initial diagnosis was progressive paralysis. He arrested and improved this degenerative collogen disease by laughing. He discovered that depression impairs the body's immunological function, and that positive emotions produce positive chemical changes (4).

O.Carl Simonton, M.D., Stephanie Matthews-Simonton, and James Creighton have spent years researching the positive effects of visualization on the eradication of cancer as supplement to orthodox medical treatment. Their clinical findings show that through the patient's self-expression of wellness (utilizing physical exercise, imagery, and art), cancer can be arrested and reversed (5).

The physical environment seems to make a difference in the recovery rate of hospitalized patients. Studies suggest that the artificiality of intensive care units, with their noisy equipment, flourescent lights, intravenous feeding and the unfamiliar faces of the medical team, traumatize the already sick person and could further impair his or her healing ability.

The Dilemma in Nursing

The dilemma facing nurses today is that many have allowed themselves to believe that pushing a button will give them a sense of professional satisfaction and self-worth. The problem is not technology itself, but the abuse of it.

If the nurse's dream is to relate to people, it goes unrealized because she is limited by the scope of machines. If her dream is to be a liaison between the patient and family, she is left in a relationship with a machine. Technology and the hospital demand that the nurse be an expert mechanic and druggist. She finds herself apathetic and exhausted with frustration. Eventually, she may quit the profession completely.

Macrobiotic health care does not foster this dependency. Through the use of palm healing, Shiatsu, diet, and compassion, the macrobiotic nurse resumes the role of her older sister, the traditional nurse. She realizes her dream.

The Macrobiotic Nurses' Guild is a newly-founded organization of professional nurses in the Boston area. We are not concerned so much about curing disease as we are in helping people to be free of the self-limitations that bring about illness. We are actively working to help people enhance the quality of their lives through their positive participation and expression of their wellness.

REFERENCES

1.   Kreiger, Delores, R.N., Ph.D., "Therapeutic Touch: Searching for Evidence of Philosophical Change." American Journal of Nursing; April 1979, pp. 660-62
2.   Ibid
3.   Quin, Janet F., R.N., M.A., "One Nurse's Evolution as a Healer." American Journal of Nursing; April 1979; pp. 662-4
4.   Macrae, Janet, R.N., M.A., "Therapeutic Touch in Illness." American Journal of Nursing; April 1979; pp. 664-5
4.   Cousins, Norman; The Anatomy of an Illness; W. W. Norton & Co., 1979
5.   Simonton, Carl O.; Matthews-Simonton, Stephanie; Creighton, James. Getting Well Again; J.P. Tarcher, Inc., Los Angeles, 1978

Macrobiotic Dietary Therapy in Belgium

Marc Van Cauwenberghe, M.D., Ghent, Belgium

The following article, reprinted from the first edition of Cancer and Diet, *is from an address at the Foundation's 1977 Cancer Conference*

I would like to make a brief report on my experiences over the last three years in recommending macrobiotics to a variety of patients. I can remember very well eight cases of cancer which I saw during this time. Generally, I divide these cases into two groups. First, are what I call "fresh" cases, in which no previous treatment has been applied, and second are those who have received previous medical treatment. The fresh cases included an older woman with skin cancer, another woman about 55 years old with breast cancer and a girl about 28 years old with a spleen disease called Vasquez's disease — I don't know if it can be called cancer, but she had a very high red blood cell count, around eight million, instead of four or five million, which is normal.

The fourth fresh case was a woman about 68 years old with cancer of the esophagus. The three first cases have all been completely cured. The first skin cancer was cured in three months and the breast cancer diappeared completely in three months. That case was finished six months ago, and since then it seems that everything is fine. The spleen disease was cured, but when the girl goes back to eating more widely, her red blood cells increase; if she stays on macrobiotic recommendations the blood level remains good.

The fourth case, the esophagus cancer, began macrobiotics about one year and a half ago. We saw her again one month and a half ago, and until that time she had been improving steadily, but recently started to have difficulty in swallowing her food. So she went back to the clinic for a checkup where they told her that probably the growth had closed the esophagus. Although she didn't want to have an operation, her family wanted her to have one because they thought she would not be able to eat therefore not survive. They did the operation and they saw that the cancer was exactly the same size as originally. There was still a passageway in the esophagus, but there was heavy inflammation of the mucus membrane so that her food had not passed through for some time. This operation was performed about a month and a half ago; they did a bypass and the tumor is still there. So we will have to continue treating this.

Then, I would like to mention four other cases: three young children with leukemia, and one lady about 60 years old with lymphosarcoma. Those four were all heavily treated with various forms of chemotherapy. So far, the three children with leukemia have died, although in one case, the family was very happy to have started macrobiotics, first of all, because the child was content; also, the child had been experiencing increasing pain and couldn't sleep, and had to sit up in bed because of difficulty in breathing. When they started the diet, after three or four days, the child slept normally and quietly and the pain disappeared. At the same time, the family was much more happy because they felt more involved with their child; they had to cook special food, the mother had to do compresses for several hours each day, etc. And even though in the end this child was not cured, the family is still very grateful that the child remained normally conscious until it died in the middle of the night, almost playing.

61

Besides these cases, with other diseases, I have also experienced that fresh cases respond more quickly to macrobiotics. Over the past three years, I have treated many cases by diet alone. Occasionally I will also use massage if I think it can help, but besides this, I haven't been using any medicine at all. I have accepted all cases who have come, and until now, have been able to manage very well any status of disease with these dietary principles according to yin and yang. However, in cases that were heavily treated, especially with cortisone therapy, the cure is much slower and sometimes can only be achieved after a couple of years. I will mention a number of diseases that I have been able to cure completely in the past three years: one bladder infection resistent to all kinds of antibiotic treatment. One case of overall body eczema. One girl, 20 years old, with acne all over her face. Several cases of heavy menstrual pain which had regularly occurred for many years. Several cases of a very long history of chronic constipation and chronic diarrhea. One case of hoarseness of the voice which the patient had experienced for one year was cured in four days through diet number seven. After four days his voice came back. The number seven diet consists generally of whole cereal grains only, with no supplements such as vegetables. This is recommended for short periods only.

I have found that if this diet is used for the right patient during a certain specified time, and the patient is regularly checked, it often results in a very quick cure. We have also cured several cases of middle ear infection in babies. A case of hay fever. One case of bifida disease for 15 years is now already half cured, half of the back is normally flexible. When he came in to see me it was completely calcified. Two cases of rheumatoid arthritis are now in the process of cure. In three months both cases have completely discontinued medication which had previously amounted to up to 20 pills a day. In both cases, the movement of the hands and all joints is slowly getting better, and also the swelling has completely gone, but still the normal movement is not there.

Further, several cases of kidney stones. It's very common that when people start macrobiotics, kidney stones dissolve and come out. Several cases of migraine. One case of bone fracture of the thigh which was cured in half of the time that was expected; in half the time the callous formation had been finished. One case of a 20-year-old benign thyroid tumor, which was broader than the head, which shrank down to two-thirds or three-fourths of its original size. At the same time, whenever this lady would walk, she experienced prolapse of the uterus. She was cured in three months just by diet, which made the tissues less watery and so she regained the original tension.

We have also experienced many cures of diabetes, especially in older patients. I would like to point out that with other dietetic approaches, of course, diabetes disappears also. But that diabetes disappears with macrobiotics is very strange, because this diet contains a large amount of carbohydrates. There is something that does not fit within the normal thinking about diabetes to explain these cures.

Besides these, many patients have come with complaints of an unknown origin, and in about 75 percent of these cases, if they started to cook and do treatments with right mental approach, they have relieved their conditions, and are now very grateful to have found out about the macrobiotic way of life.

CHAPTER THREE
Diet and Heart Disease

Diet and Heart Disease

Haruo Kushi, Harvard School of Public Health, Boston

While the focus of this book is on diet and cancer, it is important to remember that diet plays a role in the development and prevention of many other degenerative diseases. Of primary public health importance among these diseases is coronary heart disease, the number one killer in the United States and most other industrialized nations.

Coronary heart disease in all of its manifestations is the modern epidemic. Data from studies across the nation show that every fifth man and every seventeenth woman will have developed or died from coronary heart disease by age 60. Coronary heart disease currently accounts for one-half of all deaths in the United States. Over one million Americans will have heart attacks this year, and two-thirds of these people will die as a result. The impact of heart disease on the health of the nation can be measured not only in terms of morbidity and mortality, but also in economic terms: direct costs of cardiovascular disease have been estimated at $26.7 billion for 1977.

The pathological process underlying the vast majority of coronary heart disease and stroke episodes in Western nations is the development of atherosclerosis, the deposition of cholesterol-laden fatty plaques in blood vessels. Atherosclerosis results in narrowing of the arterial lumen, restricting the supply of oxygen to the affected tissue. Thus, atherosclerosis in the coronary arteries can lead to heart attacks (also called myocardial infarction), in the cerebral arteries to stroke, and in the renal arteries to kidney failure.

While the exact mechanism underlying atherogenesis — the development of these plaques — is not clearly understood, it has been hypothesized that the basic process involves injury to the endothelial cells lining the arterial walls, followed by a pouring of blood fats through this injury to lodge in the intimal space within the vessel wall. Fibrous growth may occur, resulting in the fibrous fatty plaque typical of atherosclerosis.

Many different factors can apparently lead to the initial injury of the endothelial cells. These range from high blood lipids, high blood pressure, or carboxyhemoglobin from cigarette smoke, to bacterial infections and auto-immune disorders. Because of this, it has been suggested that blood vessel injury may occur throughout the world. But in the less developed countries, this injury will usually be repaired with little or no harmful effects. It is apparently only in those nations whose populations typically have high blood lipids that atherosclerosis develops. This disease is so widespread in Western nations such as the United States that 48% of males in their early twenties already have evidence of atherosclerosis. (1)

The Role of Serum Cholesterol

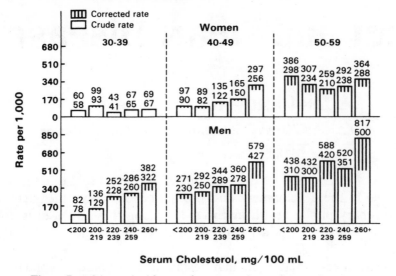

Figure 7 — *24-year incidence of coronary heart disease, by serum cholesterol level.* *(from* The Framingham Study)

The importance of high blood lipids — specifically serum cholesterol — in the development of atherosclerosis has been demonstrated beyond any reasonable doubt by many studies. The Framingham study, a prospective epidemiological study which has followed approximately five thousand men and women for over three decades, has established serum cholesterol level as one of the three most powerful risk indicators for subsequent cardiovascular disease, the other two being blood pressure and cigarette smoking (2). For example, the incidence of coronary heart disease among males was over four times greater among those with cholesterol levels above 260 mg/dl than among those with cholesterol levels below 200 mg/dl (see figure 7).

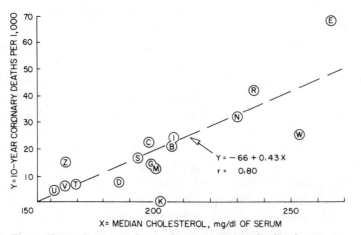

Figure 8 — *Coronary heart disease age-standardized ten-year death rates of the cohorts versus the median serum cholesterol levels (mg per dl) of the cohorts. All men judged free of coronary heart disease at entry. The coefficient of correlation is* r = 0.82. *(from Keys,* Seven Countries)

This relationship of increasing risk of coronary heart disease with increasing serum cholesterol level has been corroborated in studies in Albany, Minneapolis, and elsewhere throughout the United States and the world. One landmark study in this respect was the Seven Countries study (3) which followed over 12,000 men in different locations in Europe, the United States and Japan. The international cross-cultural comparisons again clearly show a close relationship between serum cholesterol level and coronary heart disease incidence (see figure 8).

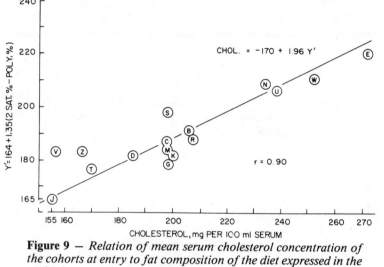

Figure 9 — *Relation of mean serum cholesterol concentration of the cohorts at entry to fat composition of the diet expressed in the multiple regression equation derived from controlled dietary experiments in Minnesota. B = Belgrade; C = Crevalcore; D = Dalmatia; E = east Finland; G = Corfu; J = Ushibuka; K = Crete; M = Montegiorgio; N = Zutphen; R = Rome railroad; S = Slavonia; T = Tanushimaru; U = American railroad; V = Velika Krsna; W = west Finland; Z = Zrenjanin.*
(from Keys, Seven Countries)

Can serum cholesterol levels be modified to decrease the coronary heart disease epidemic? The Seven Countries study has shown a strong correlation between dietary fat and serum cholesterol level (figure 9). A strong correlation between dietary saturated fat and coronary heart disease death, and between dietary saturated fat and coronary heart disease incidence has also been demonstrated (figure 10, 10A), lending support to the hypothesis that diet can influence risk of heart disease by altering serum cholesterol levels.

Diet and Serum Cholesterol

Many studies have in fact examined the effect of diet and its ability to raise or lower serum cholesterol levels. Because of the role of serum cholesterol and the nature of the fatty deposits of atherosclerosis, the dietary focus has primarily been on the effect of dietary fats and dietary cholesterol. In this regard, two studies often cited are those of Keys and co-workers (4), and of Hegsted and co-workers (5).

These studies consist of metabolic ward trials in which type of fat and amount of cholesterol were altered in the diets of persons under close observation. With each dietary change, the subsequent change in serum cholesterol level was noted. In these experiments, it was found that saturated fats such as those contained in coconut oil raise serum cholesterol levels, while polyunsaturated fats such as those that

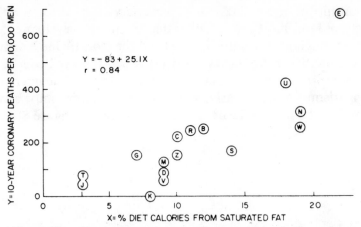

Figure 10 — *Ten-year coronary death rates of the cohorts against the percentage of dietary calories by saturated fatty acids. Cohorts as in figure 9.* *(from Keys,* Seven Countries)

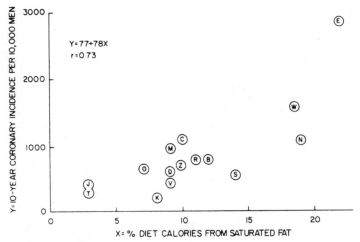

Figure 10A — *Ten-year incidence rate of coronary heart disease, by any diagnostic criterion, plotted against the percentage of dietary calories suppled by saturated fatty acids. Cohorts as in figure 9.* *(from Keys,* Seven Countries)

predominate in most vegetable oils lower serum cholesterol levels. Dietary cholesterol was found to have an effect independent of dietary fat on raising serum cholesterol (figure 11).

Investigation of non-Western or non-industrialized countries and societies also reveals a striking lack of elevated cholesterol levels and low coronary heart disease morbidity and mortality. Generally, the people in these countries also consume diets very high in complex carbohydrates, and very low in animal foods and refined sugars. A review of data from the People's Republic of China, a country with low cardiovascular disease rates, reported that the average serum cholesterol level of the population was 136 mg/dl in normal subjects, and 190 mg/dl in coronary heart disease patients (6). This compares with an average value for Americans of approximately 220 mg/dl. Even in six-year-old American children, serum cholesterol levels may average close to 190 mg/dl (7), a level which would put these children at higher than average risk of coronary heart disease in China.

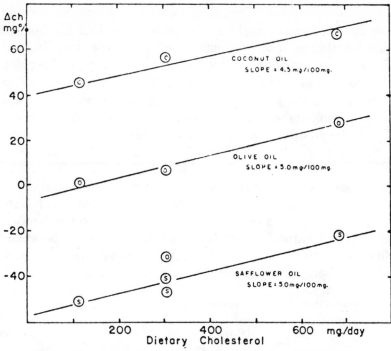

Figure 11 — *Serum cholesterol response at various levels of dietary cholesterol with three different dietary fats. Lines were drawn by inspection.* *(from Hegstead, et. al.)*

The Tarahumara Indians of Mexico, known for their long kickball games, also have very low serum cholesterol levels, averaging 125 mg/dl (8). A dietary investigation of the Tarahumaras revealed very low consumption of animal foods, the intake of which was highly corelated with serum cholesterol levels. (Table 1) This study

Correlations between the plasma cholesterol concentrations of the Tarahumara Indians and the intakes of certain foods and dietary substances[a]

Positive correlations ($P \leq 0.01$)	
Cholesterol	0.898
Animal fat	0.593
Total fat	0.552
Eggs	0.548
Animal protein	0.464
Sugar	0.323
No correlations ($P \leq 0.01$)	
Starch	0.145
Total calories	0.064
Plant sterols	0.030
Negative correlations ($P \leq 0.01$)	
Vegetable protein	−0.723
Vegetable fat	−0.403
Fiber	−0.384

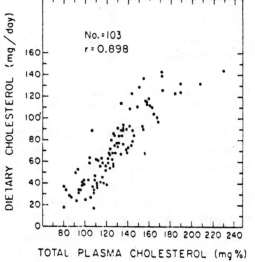

[a]Correlation coefficients were measured for a subsample of 103 adults (excluding pregnant and lactating women).

The correlation between the total plasma cholesterol and dietary cholesterol intake per day ($r = 0.898$, $P \leq 0.01$) in a subsample of the Tarahumara study.

Table 1 *(with accompanying figure). (from Connor, et. al.)*

67

was significant in that it was one of the first studies to demonstrate a strong correlation between individual dietary intake levels and individual serum cholesterol levels in a free-living population. This correlation has usually been difficult to observe because of the large amount of individual variation in food intake from day to day.

Perhaps the most interesting of these cross-cultural comparisons are the investigations comparing Japanese in Japan with Japanese in Hawaii and in California (9, 10). As with all migrant studies, these comparisons have the advantage of comparing genetically similar groups of people — in this case, all of Japanese ancestry — in different environments. Additionally, since Japan is a highly industrialized country, similar in this respect to the United States, inferences from differences in diet between these three groups can be made with more than the usual confidence. As can be seen in Table 2, the trends in comparing these three populations has shown that the Japanese in Japan eat much less fat and saturated fat, and much more complex carbohydrate than in California, with Hawaiian intakes falling between the two. This also held true for serum cholesterol levels and coronary heart disease mortality, both of which were significantly related to dietary variables.

Table 2. *Comparisons between Japanese men in Japan, Hawaii and California*

Variable	JAPAN	HAWAII	CALIFORNIA
Myocardial Infarction Incidence and Coronary Hear Disease Mortality (cases/1000person-yrs)	1.4	3.0 2.8	4.3
Serum Cholesterol (mg/dl)	181.1 ± 38.5*	218.3 ± 38.2	228.2 ± 42.2
Dietary Variables (daily intake)			
Total Fat (g)	36.6 ± 20.4	85.1 ± 38.9	94.8 ± 36.4
Saturated Fat (g)	16.0 ± 13.3	59.1 ± 32.7	66.3 ± 30.5
Cholesterol (mg)	464.1 ± 324.4	545.1 ± 316.4	533.2 ± 297.8
Simple Carbohydrate (g)	61.1 ± 37.4	91.6 ± 54.7	96.4 ± 53.9
Complex Carbohydrate (g)	278.2 ± 104.4	168.7 ± 73.7	154.9 ± 66.1
% Calories from Carbohydrate	15.1 ± 6.9	33.3 ± 9.4	37.5 ± 8.1
% Calories from Carbohydrate	63.0 ± 11.2	46.4 ± 11.0	44.2 ± 9.4

*values are mean ± standard deviation
Adapted from Robertson, et. al. (10) and Kato, et. al. (9)

Examination of groups within industrialized societies with differing dietary habits also have shown a relationship between diet, serum cholesterol, and coronary heart disease mortality. Among the most investigated of these groups are the Seventh-day Adventists. (11, 12). It has been consistently observed that the vegetarians among the Seventh-day Adventists have lower serum cholesterol levels than the omnivores among this religious group. As a whole, Seventh-day Adventists also have lower serum cholesterol levels than the general United States population, demonstrating that other factors in their lifestyle also decreases their coronary heart disease risk. A recently published report of a six-year prospective study also showed that Seventh-day Adventists living in California have lower coronary heart disease mortality rates than their fellow Californians (12). This decreased mortality was lower for the vegetarians than the non-vegetarians, significantly so in males (figure 12.)

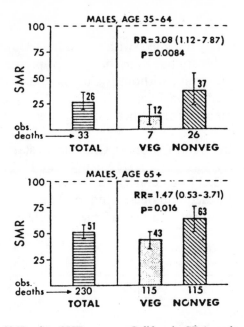

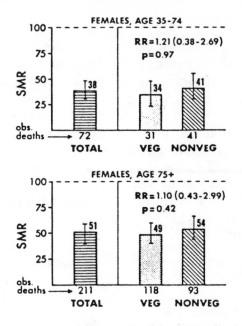

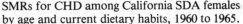

SMRs for CHD among California SDA males by age and current dietary habits, 1960 to 1965. RR = SMR in nonvegetarians/SMR in vegetarians; 95% confidence limits are shown in parentheses (18), and P *values were determined using* x^2.

SMRs for CHD among California SDA females by age and current dietary habits, 1960 to 1965.

Figure 12 - *(from Phillips, et. al.)*

Although these studies have all pointed toward a strong link between diet and coronary heart disease, none of the above studies have actually tried to alter a person's diet to see if that will lead to lower serum cholesterol levels and eventually decrease coronary heart disease morbidity and mortality. There have in fact been several clinical trials, often with persons having very high risk for coronary heart disease, which have attempted to do just that.

Table 3. *15-year follow-up in the anti-coronary club trial*

Variable	ACTIVE DIET GROUP	INACTIVE DIET GROUP	CONTROL
40-49 years			
number with hypercholesterolemia*, % change	− 50.0	− 24.9	− 5.9
coronary heart disease incidence, cases/1000 person-yrs	4.65**	12.82	7.84
50-59 years			
number with hypercholesterolemia, % change	− 44.5	− 27.4	− 13.5
coronary heart disease incidence, cases/1000 person-yrs	13.09**	18.24	20.10

* hypercholesterolemia = *serum cholesterol* ≥ 260 mg/dl
**significantly different from control, p < 0.05
Adapted from Singman, et al. (14)

Clinical Trials

Generally, these clinical trials have been classically designed, with two study groups, one given explicit instructions to change their dietary habits in the hope of preventing coronary heart disease, the other a control group, without the dietary counselling. After following these study groups for a number of years, differences between the groups in endpoints such as the proportion of coronary heart disease death and heart attack rate have been compared.

The first major clinical trial was the so-called "Anti-Coronary Club" trial, started in 1957 by the Bureau of Nutrition of the New York City Department of Health (13). It was for this study that the "Prudent Diet" was conceived, a diet with emphasis on increasing polyunsaturated fat in the diet, and decreasing total fat, saturated and cholesterol, not unlike the guidelines now known as the U.S. Dietary Goals.

Table 4. *The Los Angeles veterans administration study: eight year follow-up*

	DIET	*CONTROL*	*P*
number of men	424	422	
fatal atherosclerotic events	48	70	0.05
fatal & non-fatal atherosclerotic events	66	96	0.01
any definite or possible atherosclerotic event	110	136	0.05

Adapted from Dayton & Pearce (15)

During the course of the study, serum cholesterol levels in the group that actively followed the diet were lowered significantly relative to the control group (Table 3, 14). After fifteen years of follow-up, the incidence of coronary heart disease in the diet group was two-thirds that of the control group. A similar dietary approach was prescribed in the Los Angeles Veterans Administration study (15, 16), and again, after eight years of follow-up, the diet group had significantly less atherosclerotic events — sudden death, heart attack, or stroke — than the control group (Table 4). The diet group also had serum cholesterol levels 12.7% lower than the control group.

While the Anti-Coronary Club and Los Angeles Veterans Administration studies

Table 5. *The Oslo diet-heart study: 11-year mortality*

manifestation	*DIET*	*CONTROL*	*P*
fatal myocardial infarction	32	57	0.004
total sudden deaths	52	53	—
total coronary heart disease mortality	79	94	0.097
total cardiovascular mortality	88	102	0.13
total mortality	101	108	—
serum cholesterol at 5 years	244	285	
% decrease from initial value	17·6	3.7	

Adapted from Leren (17)

were aimed at primary prevention of atherosclerotic disease, another trial of diet and heart disease, the Oslo Diet-Heart study, (17) was aimed at secondary prevention. Thus, the study population consisted of patients with past history of heart trouble who were then followed for eleven years. Again, serum cholesterol levels in the diet group were significantly lower than that of the control group, as was the number of fatal heart attacks (Table 5). However, there was virtually no difference in total mortality between the two groups. The same effect was reported in the Finnish Mental Hospital Study, (18) in which one hospital was given a serum cholesterol lowering diet, while another hospital served as the control group (Table 6).

Table 6. *Mortality in the Finnish Mental Hospital study*

Cause	men		women	
	DIET	CONTROL	DIET	CONTROL
coronary heart disease	6.61*	14.08	5.21	7.90
cerebrovascular disease	1.74	2.42	2.23	2.02
other cardiovascular disease	3.18	2.47	3.14	2.40
cancer	5.02	3.96	4.08	3.72
all diseases	32.00	35.96	29.05	27.21
all causes	34.84	39.50	30.87	29.01

* significantly different from control, p = 0.05   Adapted from Miettinen, et. al. (18)

Unfortunately, these clinical trials have failed to be very dramatic in their effect, leading skeptics to claim that dietary prevention of heart disease has yet to be demonstrated conclusively and therefore may not be possible. However, there are two simple reasons that the effect has not been strong. The first of these is that the dietary changes were minor — it could be argued that it is remarkable that significant differences were observed with such small dietary changes. One can only speculate what might have been observed if the diet group had eaten macrobiotically rather than followed variations of the Prudent Diet. The other reason is that in these studies, the diet groups still had average serum cholesterol levels above that which is average for Americans — a level which still leads to an atheroslcerosis epidemic. Thus, the experience of the diet groups could not begin to approach the experiences of vegetarians or non-Western societies. The dietary groups were still galloping towards atherosclerosis; they only were galloping at slightly slower speeds than the controls.

Therefore, interpretation of these studies needs to be made in the context of the whole of cardiovascular research. While any one these studies has questionable significance, they have all demonstrated an impact on coronary heart disease incidence and mortality. That the impact has been in the direction predicted by other studies reinforces the conclusion that, in the aggregate, these trials are convincing evidence for the important role of diet in the prevention of coronary heart disease.

Implications for Macrobiotics

It should be stressed that although dietary fat and cholesterol have been the research emphasis when examining the effect of diet on heart disease, they are not the only dietary components that seem to affect serum cholesterol levels. Among the other factors which have been looked at are fiber (19), animal and vegetable protein (20), and type of carbohydrate (21). For all these implicated dietary factors, the macrobiotic diet is considerably more favorable for influencing serum cholesterol levels and heart disease rates than the diet of the average American. Thus, the lowest serum cholesterol values ever reported for a group living in an industrialized society were those of Boston area macrobiotic people (22).

Table 7. *Serum cholesterol and blood pressures of macrobiotic people*

Reference	number of persons	Serum Cholesterol mg/dl	Blood Pressure (mm/Hg)	
			Systolic	Diastolic
(22) Sachs et. al. N. Engl. J. Med.	115	126 ± 30* (184 ± 37)**	108 ± 12 (119 ± 11)	63 ± 10 (77 ± 8)
(23) Sacks et. al. Am. J. Epidemiol.	127 (♀) 83 (♂)		109.7 ± 11.5 100.9 ± 9.3	60.9 ± 10.8 58.2 ± 12.0
(24) Sacks et. al. J. Am. Med. Assoc.	21	140	104	60.3
(25) Bergan & Brown J. Am. Diet. Assoc.	44 (♀) 32 (♂)	148 ± 32 154 ± 30		
(26) East West Journal	11	121 range: 102-147		
(27) Wageningen Institute Netherlands	40	146 (adult, 28-40) (212) 127 (child, 6-11) (162)		

* values are mean ± standard deviation   **control values in parentheses

Listed in Table 7 are the reported values for serum cholesterol and blood pressures for macrobiotic people. It has yet to be found that the serum cholesterol values of macrobiotics approach the atherogenic levels typical of the majority of Americans. The blood pressure values are also lower than that usually observed in the American population. That these low values were due in large part to the diet of macrobiotics was demonstrated in a study soon to be published in the *Journal of the American Medical Association* (24).

In this study, twenty-one macrobiotic individuals were asked to ingest beef to examine the effect of meat on serum cholesterol levels and blood pressure. After two weeks on a macrobiotic control diet during which baseline measurements were taken, the study participants ate 250 grams of beef per day for four weeks. This meat eating period was followed by two weeks of the macrobiotic control diet. Throughout the study, serum cholesterol and blood pressure measurements were taken.

While on the meat diet, serum cholesterol levels rose from baseline values significantly, from 140 mg/dl to 166 mg/dl. Systolic blood pressure also rose significantly, by about 3 mm Hg. After returning to the macrobiotic diet, both of these increased levels fell back to baseline values, showing fairly strongly that ingestion of beef was responsible for the increase in these cardiovascular risk factors.

In addition, tentative plans are underway to examine the efficacy of the macrobiotic diet in actually promoting the regression of coronary atherosclerosis. While regression of atherosclerosis has been demonstrated in sub-human primates, (28) it has only been implied in humans, by case studies and the experience of World War II famines in Europe. If regression of coronary atherosclerosis is demonstrated, it will be the first time this has been shown in a controlled scientific setting.

Because of the extremely favorable risk factor status of macrobiotic persons, the macrobiotic diet has been considered to be perhaps the optimal diet in terms of coronary heart disease risk. While this has not yet been tested in a clinical trial or prospective study, case studies such as those following this article and the experience of patients from Pritikin's Longevity Center, where a diet similar to macrobiotics is prescribed, are encouraging. A dietary role in the development of heart disease as evidenced by the studies mentioned here show that macrobiotics, if widely practiced, could vastly diminish the health and financial burden currently exacted by coronary heart disease and related cardiovascular disorders.

Addendum

It should be noted that although this review has focused on the role in altering serum cholesterol levels, there is also some evidence that diet can favorably alter blood pressure levels, a major heart disease risk factor along with serum cholesterol and cigarette smoking. This is supported by the low blood pressures of macrobiotic people as seen in Table 7.

It should also be noted that coronary heart disease is a multi-factorial disease, and that diet is only one of many factors that influence the probability of developing this disease. Cigarette smoking is the third leg of the cardiovascular risk factor triad as described by the Framingham study, but is just one of several factors involved. Other potential risk factors include the presence of diabetes — which may also be related in part to diet — and the role of physical activity in preventing coronary heart disease. Persons with compulsive behavior as opposed to a more relaxed attitude also have a greater risk of heart disease. Obesity is a practical risk factor, as it is usually accompanied by elevated serum cholesterol, elevated blood pressure, or onset of diabetes.

However, the multi-factorial nature of heart disease should not be used as an excuse to minimize the importance of diet in the development of this disease. Changing one's diet can be the first step toward taking responsibility for one's own life and making lifestyle changes for better health, physical and otherwise.

REFERENCES

1. McNamara JJ, Molot MA, Stremple JT, et. al.: Coronary artery disease in combat casualties in Vietnam. J. Am. Med. Assoc. *216*:1185-7, 1971.
2. Dawber TR: *The Framingham Study: The Epidemiology of Atherosclerotic Disease*. Harvard University Press, Cambridge MA, 1980.
3. Keys A: *Seven Countries: A Multivariate Analysis of Death and Coronary Heart Disease*. Harvard University Press, Cambridge MA, 1980.
4. Keys A, Anderson JT, Grande F: Serum cholesterol response to changes in the diet. I-IV. Metabolism *14*:747-787, 1965.
5. Hegsted DM, McGandy RB, Myers ML, Stare FJ: Quantitative effects of dietary fat on serum cholesterol in man. Am. J. Clin. Nutr. *17*(11): 281-295, 1965.
6. Van die Redaskie: Coronary heart disease in China. South African Med. J. *47*:1485, 1973.

7. Crawford PB, Clark MJ, Pearson RL, Huenemann RL: Serum cholesterol of 6-year-olds in relation to environmental factors. J. Am. Diet. Assoc. *78*(1):41-46, 1981.

8. Connor WE, Cerqueira MT, Connor RW, et. al.: The plasma lipids, lipoproteins, and diet of the Tarahumara Indians of Mexico. Am. J. Clin. Nutr. *31*(7):1131-1142, Jul 1978.

9. Kato H, Tillotson J, Nichaman MZ, et. al.: Epidemiologic studies of coronary heart disease and stroke in Japanese men living in Japan, Hawaii and California: Serum lipids and diet. Am. J. Epidemiol. *97*(6):372-385, 1973.

10. Robertson TL, Kato H, Rhoads GG, et. al.: Epidemiologic studies of coronary heart disease and stroke in Japanese men living in Japan, Hawaii and California: Incidence of myocardial infarction and death from coronary heart disease. Am. J. Cardiol. *39*(2):239-243, Feb 1977.

11. West RO, Hayes OB: Diet and serum cholesterol levels: a comparison between vegetarians and nonvegetarians in a Seventh-day Adventist group. Am. J. Clin. Nutr. *21*(8):853-862, Aug 1968.

12. Phillips RL, Lemon FR, Beeson WL, Kuzma JW: Coronary heart disease mortality among Seventh-day Adventists with differing dietary habits: a preliminary report. Am. J. Clin. Nutr. *31*(10):S191-S198, Oct 1978.

13. Christakis G, Rinzler SH, Archer M, et. al.: The Anti-Coronary Club: A dietary approach to the prevention of coronary heart disease — a seven-year report. Am. J. Publ. Health *56*(2):299-314, Feb 66.

14. Singman HS, Berman SN, Cowell C, et. al.: The Anti-Coronary Club: 1957 to 1972. Am. J. Clin. Nutr. *33*(6):1183-1191, Jun 1980.

15. Dayton S, Pearce ML: Prevention of coronary heart disease and other complications of atherosclerosis by modified diet. Am. J. Med. *46*:751-762, May 1969.

16. Dayton S, Pearce ML, Hashimoto S, et. al.: A clinical trial of high unsaturated fat diet. Circulation *39-40*(Suppl. 2):1, Jul 1969.

17. Leren P: The Oslo Diet-Heart study: Eleven-year report. Circulation *42*:935-942, Nov 1970.

18. Miettinen M. Turpeinen O, Karvonen MJ, et. al.: Effect of cholesterol-lowering diet on mortality from coronary heart-disease and other causes: A twelve-year clinical trial in men and women. Lancet *2*:835-838, 21 Oct 1972.

19. Kritchevsky D: Dietary fiber and other dietary factors in hypercholesterolemia. Am. J. Clin. Nutr. *30*(6):979-984, Jun 1977.

20. Sirtori CR, Agradi E, Conti F, et. al.: Soybean protein diet in the treatment of type II hyperlipoproteinemia. Lancet *1*:275, 1977.

21. Reiser S, Hallfrisch J, Michaelis OE, et. al.: Isocaloric exchange of dietary starch and sucrose in humans. I. Effects on levels of fasting blood lipids. Am. J. Clin. Nutr. *32*:1659-1669, 1978.

22. Sacks FM, Castelli WP, Donner A, Kass EH: Plasma lipids and lipoproteins in vegetarians and controls. N. Engl. J. Med. *292*:1148-1151, 1975.

23. Sacks FM, Rosner B, Kass EH: Blood pressure in vegetarians. Am. J. Epidemiol. *100*:390-398, 1974.

24. Sacks FM, Donner A, Castelli WP, et. al.: Effect of ingestion of meat on plasma cholesterol of vegetarians. J. Am. Med. Assoc. (in press), 1981.

25. Bergan JG, Brown PT: Nutritional status of "new" vegetarians. J. Am. Diet. Assoc. *76*(2):151-155, Feb 1980.

26. Monte T: The Staff of Life. East West Journal *10*(11):47, Nov 1980.

27. Vermuyten R: Private Communication.

28. Armstrong ML, Warner ED, Connor WE: Regression of coronary atheromatosis in rhesus monkeys. Circulation Res. *27*:59-67, Jul 1970.

Macrobiotics and Heart Disease

Michio Kushi, East West Foundation, Boston

The following article is reprinted from the November, 1980 East West Journal.

Before we can cure ourselves of this sickness, or of any illness for that matter, the first thing each of us must do is deeply reflect upon our lives. We must ask ourselves: Is my daily food making my health stronger or is it contributing to my illness? Also, if we are employed in an office in which we spend most of the day sitting at a desk, we should ask ourselves if there is a balance between our mental and physical activity. Am I living an active, happy life, or is my life sedentary and stagnated?

If we want to be healthy, active, and happy, we need to change our way of eating and seek out more activity.

We know that diet is the underlying cause and the overriding cure of heart disease. Many people with cardiovascular problems have changed their way of eating and activity and had their health restored. In order to successfully treat heart disease, it is best to reduce the intake of the foods high in saturated fat and cholesterol,[1] including red meat, eggs and dairy products, as well as refined grains, synthetic chemicals, and refined sugar. In their place, it is advisable to eat 50 to 60 percent whole grains (brown rice, wheat, barley, millet, rye, corn, and others); 25 percent locally grown, cooked vegetables; 10 percent beans and sea vegetables; the rest of our diet is made up of fish (if desired), soups (miso and shoyu broth, particularly), local fruits, some seeds, nuts, and certain condiments. This is the standard macrobiotic diet (please see Chapter I).

This diet will help the body to discharge toxins and fat deposits that have built up over the years, usually since before a person was a teenager.[2]

Modifications in the Standard Diet

The standard diet can be altered slightly based on the individual's needs and state of health. Basically, there are two types of heart disease: one is the result of foods high in fat and cholesterol. This results in hardening of the arteries and fat deposits surrounding the heart. The heart and arteries lose their elasticity

---

[1]Cholesterol, a sterol, is a fatlike substance most of which is manufactured by the liver. Cholesterol is involved in synthesizing sex hormones and transporting essential fatty acids through the blood to other cells in the body. It also serves as part of the covering of nerve cells. The body produces all the cholesterol a person needs; however, scientists have determined that the average American each day takes in about 600 mg. through his or her food. Little wonder, then, that the average American has a cholesterol level of 250 mg. and above. These levels put a great number of Americans in the "high risk" category for heart attack and stroke as well as contribute to a lower quality of life in the incidences of hypertension, lethargy, and overweight.

[2]In September, 1980, eleven *East West Journal* members had their blood cholesterol levels measured. The attendant at the Beacon Labs in Boston took a small vial of blood from each person and the results came in a few hours later. The tests showed that the average blood cholesterol level at the *Journal* was 121 milligrams. The cholesterol levels ranged from a high of 147 mg. to a low of 102 mg. Most of the eleven staff members were under 115 mg. The average age among the eleven people was 30. All have been eating a grain- and vegetable-centered diet for at least two years. Moreover, all eleven come from middle-class backgrounds and grew up on the typical modern diet of meat, dairy foods, and sugar before taking up whole foods.

and vitality, and the heart labors excessively in order to do its job of pumping blood throughout the body. The fat and cholesterol that collects in the arteries reduce blood and oxygen to the heart and brain. Eventually, enough of these fatty deposits build up and cause a heart attack or stroke. This condition, we may say, is very yang — contracted and hardened: the arteries are blocked by the fat and cholesterol that has built up.

The second type of heart disease is a condition that arises from drinking too many liquids, particularly alcohol, soda pop, caffeinated beverages, fruit juices, and eating too many refined foods, sugar, and fruits. This type of sickness we can refer to as a more yin condition; the heart is swollen, it beats irregularly, and is weak.

To treat the yang, contracted condition, we can begin reducing the foods mentioned earlier, especially foods high in saturated fat and cholesterol. We can eat the standard macrobiotic diet and also provide some good quality yin foods in order to bring the heart back into a state of balance. Balance is an equilibrium between yin and yang, between expansion and contraction.

For a person with a more yang condition, the cooking can be lighter, such as steamed and lightly boiled vegetables. Salads and raw vegetables are fine in moderate amounts. Locally grown fruit and fruit juice occasionally are also good for this condition. These are examples of good quality yin foods. Less miso and natural shoyu may be used in soup; the soup should have only a mild flavor. Wakame seaweed and some vegetables can also be included in the soup stock.

Beans, especially adukis, chickpeas, and lentils, are also encouraged. Hard leafy green vegetables are an excellent source of fiber and very effective in helping the body discharge excess fat which has accumulated in the intestines and elsewhere.

For a yin condition in which the heart is swollen, weak, and beats irregularly, we recommend the standard macrobiotic diet. At the same time, we recommend including more good quality yang foods. The cooking can be longer, and the grains we eat — 50 to 60 percent of our daily intake of food — are usually pressure-cooked. Miso soup and shoyu broth can be a little stronger, and fish can be included as a regular dish. When we eat fish, the portions should be small, and a little grated ginger can be used. Ginger helps digest any oils that may be used in cooking. Whole grains are always our principal foods, even if fish is served with the meal.

Condiments and Special Dishes

For many thousands of years, traditional cultures recognized the importance of natural foods, condiments, and medicines made of natural ingredients. In ancient times, there were no pharmaceutical companies to dispense drugs; so through trial and error and an understanding of nature, ancient people discovered many natural remedies for sickness. Of course, diet is our principal means of preventing and reversing illness. However, traditional people discovered remedies which speed recovery through the unique properties of certain plants and food combinations. Many of these remedies are put down in writing in the ancient text, *The Yellow Emperor's Classic of Internal Medicine,* the oldest medical book in the world, dating back to about 2600 B.C. I encourage everyone to read and study this great work.

There are several important medicinal preparations and condiments effective in the therapy of heart disease. For those who suffer from both yang and yin heart conditions, macrobiotic condiments such as gomosio, tekka, roasted wakame seaweed, and umeboshi plums are very helpful. Gomasio has been found to be particularly effective in restoring elasticity to the heart.

For a yang, contracted condition in which a great deal of saturated fat, cholesterol, and salt have been eaten in the past, it is better to use condiments sparingly and increase vegetables such as daikon radish, which helps dissolve fat deposits in the arteries and heart. When cooking daikon — either boiling or steaming — a few drops of shoyu can be used. Scallions and spring onions, used as a garnish or cooked into soups, are also helpful. Shiitake mushrooms, used to make a soup stock or cooked in soup, are useful in discharging animal fats. Kombu tea, which is kombu seaweed boiled in water, or kombu powder dissolved in boiling water, and pearl barley, if it can be obtained, are both very effective at dissolving fat deposits in the body. Pearl barley can be pressure-cooked or boiled in the same way as other grains or roasted and ground up to be used as a tea with boiling water. Corn is also an excellent grain for the heart, very strengthening. Watercress and carrot tops cooked together help to restore elasticity to arteries as does seitan cooked with a little salt. Ginger juice, added to miso soup — but not boiled — is helpful in breaking up fats.

Those with a yin, swollen heart can use the condiments mentioned earlier. In addition, ranshio can be taken once a day for three days - no more (see page 39). This strengthens the heart and stimulates beating. In traditional Japan - where there was virtually no cardiovascular disease - when children would prepare to run races, their mothers would often secretly given them ranshio to make their hearts stronger and therefore help them to run faster.

Another ancient remedy for a yin condition is ume-sho-bancha tea, which also aids in the strengthening of the heart. For this tea, umeboshi plum is mixed with shoyu and then hot bancha tea is added. The order is very important; otherwise the tea will have little or no effect.

Dandelion tea, in which the stem, leaves, and roots of the dandelion (the flower is not used) are mixed with boiling water, can be drunk daily for a yin condition; it is very good for strengthening the heart. One last tea is bancha-shoyu tea, in which bancha twig tea is added to a few drops of natural shoyu. This creates a more alkaline blood condition, which is fundamental to health.

Blood Quality

When we are healthy, our blood — which is slightly saline — is in an alkaline condition. Fermented products, such as miso and natural shoyu, help keep the blood in an alkaline state, thus keeping our overall condition healthy. When we eat such foods as refined sugar, too much fruit or fruit juices, and red meat and dairy products, our blood becomes acidic and the result is that we are prone to more illnesses. Sickness — germs — thrive in acidic blood.

By eating foods high in saturated fat, cholesterol, artificial chemicals, refined sugar, and other unhealthful products, other organs, whose job it is to cleanse the blood, are overworked. If we continue to eat this way, the organs are worked to capacity but still cannot fully eliminate such elements from our system. The result is unhealthy blood and weak, tired organs. When our kidneys, liver, spleen, and lungs are unable to cleanse our blood, our hearts suffer all the more. More fat builds up around the heart and in the arteries. The heart, like other organs, must labor excessively. You can see that when we are in this condition, our health is quickly declining.

A New Approach to Life and Health

There are many reasons why modern medicine has developed a more fragmented view of life and health. One reason is that modern anatomy has measured the size and location of the heart and other organs but has not yet discovered the overall dynamic function of these organs in relationship to each other and to the cosmos. The reason for this is that present day anatomy draws most of its knowledge from autopsies rather than living organisms. Of course, when the body is dead, there isn't much going on inside besides decay. However, during a person's life, all of our organs are working in concert with each other. Thus, in order to strengthen the heart, we need to strengthen the kidneys, liver, spleen, pancreas, and lungs — all organs — since the healthy functioning of the heart depends on the healthy functioning of our entire system.

The rhythmic beating of the heart is one of nature's most beautiful expressions of yang and yin, contracting and expanding more than 100,000 times a day, three billion times in a lifetime.

In the *Gospel According to Thomas,* Jesus says, "If they ask you, 'What is the sign of your Father in you?' say to them: 'It is a movement and a rest.'" The heart is a perfect metaphor for the expression of God, the Order of the Universe, within each of us. In order to preserve the health of this organ, we must preserve a balance between yin and yang, between expansion and contraction.

CHAPTER FOUR
Case Histories (Cancer and Cancer Related)*

Metastatic Prostate Cancer

Irving Malow, Evanston, Illinois, 1981
Contributed by Keith Block, M.D.

A 60-year-old caucasian gentleman, Mr. Irving Malow, visited my office on 9/24/80 virtually riddled with cancerous lessions on the spine, pelvis, and shoulders; secondary to his earlier diagnosis of prostate cancer. Mr. Malow experienced his initial symptoms and diagnosis in 1975. His disease process progressed from that time with a steady deterioration of his health. Prior conventional therapy had included a partial orchiectomy, radiation therapy, and chemotherapy consisting of adriamycin, cytoxan, and cis-platinum. He stopped cytoxan and adriamycin after three treatments and stopped cis-platinum after one quarter of the treatment. During his regimen of cis-platinum chemotherapy, Mr. Malow threw up several times every hour for the following twelve hours until quitting the treatment. Further recommendations for chemotherapy were answered by Mr. Malow's firm statement: "I refuse to go on with these debilitating and torturous treatments."

During the time of his visit he expressed a definitive opinion refusing "under any circumstances" further chemotherapy (due to previous ill side-effects) other than the hormone stilbesterol. (Note: Mr. Malow had reduced his stilbesterol dosage by 50% just four weeks after initiation of the macrobiotic diet and reduced this still further to a quarter of his original dosage by his own volition from 1/8 to 1/16 of the original dosage and finally went off this medication completely.)

While practicing the prescribed macrobiotic dietary program, Mr. Malow's appetite returned, his pain ceased, and his energy level increased. Mr. Malow attributes his pain relief totally to the macrobiotic diet. (This has now been substantiated in other cases that have been relieved of severe spinal pain just several weeks following initiation of the macrobiotic regimen.)

With confirmed return to well being and improved activity, the patient elected to proceed with diagnostic bone scans. Radiologists at Weiss Memorial Hospital in Chicago found the patient's scans to be markedly improved, and an expert at St. Francis Hospital in Evanston, Illinois, found the recent scans to be "grossly normal." (Note: Upon discussion with numerous oncologists in the Evanston/ Chicago area, the general opinion was that hormonal therapy would not be a likely explanation for the reversal in Mr. Malow's bone scan.)

The care and improvement seen with this patient, as well as others presently on the same regimen and suffering from metastatic prostate cancer, makes it imperative that serious investigations of this approach be viewed by the medical community without delay.

As President Edward Scanlon of the ACS begins a 6-year study to determine lifestyle effects on cancer development, I urge the general public not to wait for the obvious results. There is a pressing need to promptly change not only our dietary habits, but our lifestyles as well. By introducing the macrobiotic approach to health care, we can look forward to a new profile of well being for the American people.

Below, Mr. Malow exemplifies the feelings of several thousand people, who have begun the battle against terminal thinking patterns:

"When I was told I had cancer six years ago, I literally brainwashed myself, refusing to accept the fact that the cancer would overwhelm me. I simply referred to it as my 'little cancer' since I wanted to make it a lesser important evil, rather than a strong all-encompassing, incurable problem. I was told by friends and doctors alike that my positive mental attitude would probably have a great effect regarding the problem of cancer.

"When some friends came across the article by Dr. Sattilaro in the *Saturday Evening Post* regarding his overcoming the very same problems that I have incurred,[1] I proceeded without delay to study and follow the macrobiotic way of life. I am totally convinced that we are what we eat and that we literally destroy our bodies with the poor quality of foods, confections, etc., which we consume. When we analyze the intricate and amazing functions of our body and organs, I further decided we truly should consider the body to be a shrine, which must be given proper nourishment and care.

"At age 60, despite radiation treatment, some chemotherapy, and other minor problems associated with cancer, I continue to work full time, and also often spend some evening hours doing work. I endeavor to maintain a reasonable amount of exercise and continue to look upon cancer as something that we can overcome with diet and determination. Our amazing bodies apparently can heal themselves if we furnish the body with the proper nourishment, and eliminate that which is harmful."

See following page for Mr. Malow's bone scans.

---

[1] "An M.D. Who Conquered His Cancer," by Tom Monte, *Saturday Evening Post*, September, 1980.

Slide Reproductions of Irving Malow's Bone Scans
taken 4/24/79 and 3/3/81.

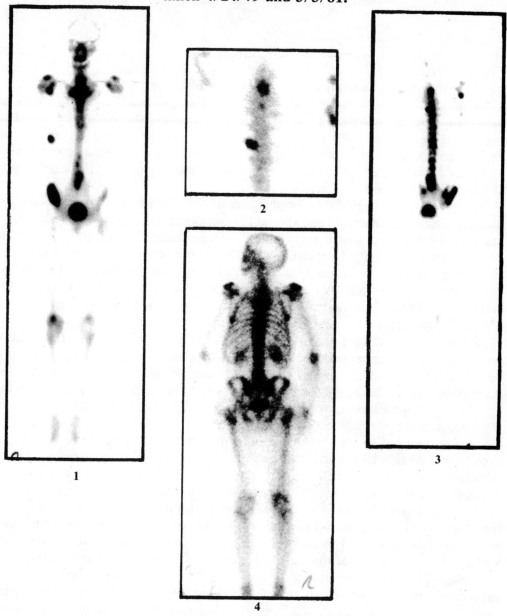

1 - This Anterior view total body scan from 4/24/79 shows extensive bone metastases (spread of cancer seen by blackened areas) with involvement to the entire right ilium (hip), the low lumbar spine, the upper thoracic spine and the right shoulder. (Note: Blackened right rib was consistent with prior fracture.)

2 -This Posterior view of the patient's upper thorax shows a close up of two metastatic areas to the thoracic spine and one area to the right shoulder.

3 - This Posterior scan from 4/24/79 shows similar metastatic spread as slide #1 of this series.

4 - This Posterior bone scan (one of a series) was taken on 3/3/81, five months following initiation of the Macrobiotic regimen. This was read as "grossly normal." There is obvious clearing of the right ilium (hip), right shoulder, and lumbar and thoracic spine.

Cervical Cancer

Donna Gail, Jamaica Plain, Massachusetts, 1981

On April 20, 1942, I was born in New Haven, Connecticut. I am now a Licensed Practical Nurse (LPN), and have been a diet consultant in California, an owner/manager of a futon business, and a macrobiotic cooking teacher.

I was raised in New Haven with four other siblings. Our family ate plenty of meat, and for us that meant beef. I was also bottle fed. My mother tried to breastfeed me, but was told she had too little milk, so she obeyed her doctor and resorted to bottle feeding. I was brought up in a small city in a housing development and was educated in Catholic schools for the most part. In nursing I worked mostly in psychiatry, and also in obstetrics.

In 1969 it was discovered that I had cancer of the cervix in situ (*in situ* means the beginning stages of cancer.) I had several Pap smears and at least two biopsies done, and for treatment and diagnosis my doctors also performed a conization at the Yale New Haven Community Hospital. Conization is the scraping of several layers of tissue all around the cervix, used for both diagnosis and treatment. The doctors had hoped that the cancer cells would be removed from my body and that would be the end of my sickness. This was not the case, however, and the cancer cells reappeared. There were no other treatments besides conization and biopsies.

At that point, I changed doctors because I wasn't happy with the one I'd had. For one thing, he recommended that I continue with the birth control pills I had just begun, and that didn't seem right to me; so I switched to an older doctor who was more conservative. Because of my young age, he decided that we would watch the condition through Pap smears every three months. The Pap smears continued coming back positive.

It never occurred to me that diet could cure cancer, but I was interested in improving my health in general. Specifically, I was interested in weight control. Although I was not fat, I had a tendency to go in that direction. So, at that time I changed my diet quite a bit, reducing my food intake in general. Specifically, I reduced my animal food intake (including dairy foods) by about one third. I reduced my intake of chemicals drastically and reduced refined flour, sugar and other sweets by 75% or more. I reduced my fat and oil consumption dramatically. Previously, I would go out of my way to eat animal fat when other people left it on their plate. I just about eliminated all canned and processed foods. Before this, my favorite foods had been frozen sweets (including ice cream, frozen cakes, frozen candy bars), beef, macaroni, salt, tomato sauce and cheese. I also cut down on alcohol, but didn't eliminate it. I still drank a lot of coffee, around 20 cups a day. I increased my fresh food intake tenfold at least; prior to this I had eaten very few vegetables.

It was about a year later that I was introduced to macrobiotics. I went to a lecture by Michio Kushi in Rhode Island in 1972. The next day I changed over to macrobiotics, making grains a major part of my diet. I took little raw food, eliminated meat and dairy products altogether, and completely eliminated strong sweets. By this time I had already eliminated coffee and alcohol from my diet. My diet became more balanced; I now had a principle to follow. That was very important because I had never had any dietary principle, nor had I understood the idea of balance.

Within six months after changing my diet, the Pap smears started coming back negative. When I tried to talk to the doctor about the fact that the cancer cells had disappeared, and he responded with "spontaneous remission."

The only thing I had changed was my diet! The conization hadn't worked; the cancer cells had appeared again after that had been done. Now, after twelve years there has still been no sign of the cancer cells reappearing.

In 1975 I went through a very stressful situation. My diet got a little loose, my eating habits became irregular and the Pap smear came back Class 4. I went to the hospital, had a repeat Pap smear, and the head of gynecology said "We have to do a biopsy. I am almost 100% sure you have cancer, and you need to have your reproductive organs removed." I went back the next day expecting him to tell me I had cancer once again. He said "No, you absolutely do not have cancer. You have an irritation. However, I still highly recommend that you have all of your organs removed as a preventive measure." I was relieved, angry and shocked, as were my family and friends. I continued to watch my Pap smears and they gradually got better, from Class 4 to Class 2. In the meantime I had a consultation with Michio Kushi, who suggested I was eating too many flour products.

Now I understand the situation more clearly. I think flour products took the place of dairy products in my diet, and affected my body in a similar way. So I gradually reduced flour products, and the Pap smears became completely negative (Class 1) by 1980.

Other Improvements

Before macrobiotics I was emotionally somewhat unstable and was diagnosed as having hypoglycemia. I was sleeping 12 hours a day and taking a nap in the afternoon. I was awakening every morning feeling more tired than when I went to sleep, and my whole body, muscles, and joints were sore every morning. I was fainting fairly often — once or twice a week. I even went to the hospital to be checked because this seemed so strange. I had the symptoms of having a heart attack with pain in chest radiating down the left arm. I had pain in my lower right quadrant area. Walking two blocks would exhaust me. I felt emotionally out of control, I would cry and get angry for no apparent reason. Finally I realized that I was behaving like the patients I had cared for in the psychiatric hospital.

It was after I changed to macrobiotics that all of these symptoms changed. I had much more energy, slept less, had much more emotional stability. The chest pains also went away, and there was no fainting.

Before macrobiotics my menstrual cycle had always been fairly regular, but was debilitatingly painful; I usually had a heavy flow for seven days. After two months of macrobiotic eating all menstrual pain disappeared; the flow was lighter and decreased to five days. I had no more bloating before my period or soreness in my breasts. I had also had problems with my ankles, such as swelling during the summer; again, within a couple of months of macrobiotic eating, those symptoms disappeared.

I also had a history of lower back trouble that would chronically incapacitate me; this lessened about 80% after the change to macrobiotics. I also used to experience tremendous pain in my ears whenever descending from a high altitude; often on airplane flights this would be so painful that I wanted to jump out the window. That also disappeared after a few months of eating macrobiotically.

My tendency towards overweight pretty much disappeared, so that I am no longer obsessed with weight control! My body has changed, too — it has become more soft, feminine and graceful.

I had had a condition similar to psoriasis since I was a child. The scales on my scalp would sometimes be the size of a quarter, a symptom common in our family. Since I started macrobiotics, that condition has disappeared. I always had about 20 pimples on the right side of my lower jaw, and they disappeared too.

I also had hemorrhoids before macrobiotics and they disappeared within a couple of months, as did my constant stuffy nose. I could not breathe through my nose and had had an operation for what was thought to be a deviated septum. After the operation I still couldn't breathe, and the doctor said my condition must be due to an allergy. After eating macrobiotically for a few months, my breathing became nearly normal.

One of the most important changes I have been able to make since becoming macrobiotic involves my relationship with my father. Up until 2 years ago, I hadn't spoken with him since I was 12 years old. Now we communicate regularly, and have discovered a great mutual respect and caring for one another.

Since I have been studying and practicing macrobiotics, I also feel much more able to help other people. As a nurse, I have found macrobiotics to be an invaluable way to assist other people to make positive changes in their lives. It has been very exciting for me to work with clients and observe the changes they have made for themselves. Much of this experience came when I was working in California for a holistic health and nutrition clinic, as a nurse practicing "diet transition guidance;" in this capacity, I was able to offer assistance and support in every aspect of a client's change from consultations and practical classes to shopping and cooking. The basis for all this work, and the ability to understand and reach people, has come from my study of the principles and practice of macrobiotics.

A nurse is naturally in a very good position to teach patients how to take care of themselves, and develop responsibility for their own health. Unfortunately, this is exactly what is not being done in most nursing today — actually, a good deal of valuable information is withheld, and further dependence is actually encouraged and perpetuated. Instead of so much time being spent on learning how to use drugs, I would like to see nurses learn more about teaching what patients can do for themselves, particularly in the area of macrobiotic, natural treatments. I think that nutrition and the link between diet and disease should become an integral part of nursing training. My own experience has shown me that this is just one more of the many wonderful things macrobiotics has to offer us today.

Granular Myoblastoma On The Vocal Cord

*Laura Anne Fitzpatrick, with
Mrs. Phyllis Fitzpatrick, Sherborn,
Massachusetts, 1981*

Laura: It was in the spring of 1979 that I was diagnosed as having a tumor on the vocal cords after my voice was getting raspy. I had tried out for cheerleading at my high school and had to tell my friends to be patient because I couldn't use my voice. That summer, in August, I had an operation on my throat in which the tumor was removed.

Mrs. Fitzpatrick: Laura's voice had completely left her. I simply felt she had been using her voice too much. We finally took her to the doctor who discovered a node on her vocal cords, recommending that she have an operation. A tumor was found, and we had to wait a few days to discover whether or not it was malignant. It turned out to be granular myoblastoma, a rare type of benign tumor. In fact, Laura's case was the only one where the tumor was on the vocal cord.

In January, 1980 we went to see a surgeon at Boston's University Hospital who specialized in laser beam surgery. It was discovered that the tumor had definitely returned following its removal in August. After the second operation, the doctor was quite sure that the laser surgery was successful and that the tumor was gone.

However, Laura's voice temporarily left her after the second operation, and during the four-week checkup following surgery, the doctor was not pleased with what he saw, since the tumor seemed to be returning. He did not want to discourage us completely, but he said that there was definite swelling. He advised Laura to return every three months for close monitoring.

In February, 1980, we saw a television program featuring Professor Jean Kohler describing his recovery from pancreatic cancer through macrobiotics. At that time we signed up for a three-day *Cancer and Diet* seminar offered through the East West Foundation. At first, my husband John and I felt uncomfortable because we saw many people who seemed to be very ill. When Michio Kushi entered, however, a comfort and calm came over me, and I began to feel very much at home. Mr. Kushi opened the seminar with a warm welcome and said "How many people here have cancer?" Among the young and old people in the room, half of the hands were raised. I was impressed by his relaxed and sensible approach, and the simplicity of his presentation. At the end of those three days, I tried to digest all of my notes. Laura, who had not attended the workshop, felt the excitement that John and I felt about the information gained during the weekend.

We called Michio Kushi to make an appointment. He told Laura that this would be very simple—to not be at all discouraged. He could support her recovery by recommending "a very simple diet."

Laura: We began to introduce this way of eating to our family, and with two sisters and three brothers still at home, this became quite an adventure. We cleaned out the cupboards and moved the remaining food to another section. I just loved

87

the food. We invited an experienced macrobiotic cook to come into our home to prepare the food, and it was delicious to me from the very beginning. My 11-year-old brother's first question was "What do you do on birthdays?" He knew that this would be a change, but he was concerned that the change would be forever, and that he would no longer enjoy his meals. My sisters immediately went on the diet.

Mrs. Fitzpatrick: John and I both wanted to support Laura, and we also began to eat in this new way as much as we could. We changed our stove from electric to gas, and the adventures continued as we truly tried to understand the principles behind the diet. Laura temporarily went on a more restricted diet which did not include oil. She also went to bed with taro potato plasters wrapped around her neck.

Laura: I experienced may changes throughout my body because toxins were being released rapidly. As a result I felt a great deal more energy, though my voice was still raspy and weak. I was going to a special therapist who was teaching me to express myself despite the weakness of my voice.

As I continued with the diet, however, my voice definitely started improving, becoming less raspy. We were noticing changes that were taking place, but were concentrating on the diet rather than the tumor.

In early spring, when we met with the doctor, I was shocked to find that no operation was necessary. There was still scar tissue from the first operation but my condition was greatly improved. The doctor suggested that we check on my condition every three months.

Mrs. Fitzpatrick: Laura's condition continued to improve through the fall. Every three months she returned to the doctor who found that her condition remained stable. There was no suggestion of further surgery.

Laura: In November, I started to deviate from the recommended diet. I began cooking with oil, ate turkey at Thanksgiving, and continued in this way until Christmas, 1980. Symptoms started to return during that time, for example, my voice grew weak and continually got worse. We went back for a checkup with the doctor, although I knew that I was the one who was controlling my situation or pushing it out of control. When the doctor saw me, he said that the tumor was again large and had to be operated on immediately. This was in January of 1981. I cried and immediately understood what the problem was. At that point we asked for a two-month reprieve. The doctor consented, saying that two months wasn't that crucial, especially after we explained that the diet had been helping my condition and that we understood what was happening. We immediately called Michio Kushi.

Mrs. Fitzpatrick: He looked at Laura and immediately saw that she had been cheating.

Laura: He scolded me humorously, and I decided I was ready to get back to basics and resume the diet he had recommended.

Mrs. Fitzpatrick: This experience brought home how difficult it was for Laura to practice the diet in the middle of her active life. Other people didn't understand the situation. For example, college attendance is very difficult because dormitories and cafeterias tend not to encourage a more natural diet and way of life. Support of family and friends is such an important part of maintaining balance. I will be meeting soon with the staff at the university Laura is attending to strongly request that they establish a program in the school to support a more natural way of eating and living.

Laura: At this point, Michio recommended that I be even more careful with my diet for two months, so that my return to the doctor would be successful. I again began to discharge a lot of mucus and felt a tremendous cleansing coming very rapidly. I resumed the taro potato compresses each night. One humorous sidelight of this was that my father's T-shirts were disappearing, and he would find them with mysterious brown spots from the remains of the taro potato. I found that whenever I missed the ginger and taro potato plaster compress for a few days, the mucus would not discharge as freely. I prepared all the compresses by myself and the routine became normal. We maintained our sense of humor during this period, and the family would often joke about the daily events.

In March I spent two weeks as a guest at the Kushi house. Everyone in the house was so warm and helpful, and special breakfasts and lunches were prepared for me to eat during my school days. We returned to the doctor in June, following this two-month practice, and he was again surprised at the incredible progress I had made. I would see one of two doctors every three months, and they were maintaining contact with each other to monitor my progress. One is on the staff of the Leonard Morse Hospital, and the other is with the Boston University Hospital. The doctor at Leonard Morse saw that the tumor was in a very stable, improved condition, and that we again had nothing to worry about. In three months, I will again return for a checkup.

I learned from this experience that the diet makes sense. I know that it is my responsibility to maintain this way of life. I have learned a lot about myself and have gained a great deal of confidence from this experience.

Mrs. Fitzpatrick: I feel that Laura has grown considerably during this past year. I strongly believe that negative situations can create positive results, provided that attitude and practice work together. It's most important that a person facing a negative situation does not give up. Rather, it's important to open your eyes and gain confidence that something will come along that will work. We were very fortunate to have found this way of life before it became too late. If Laura had had more operations, her voice would have continued to grow worse. Macrobiotics gave her the opportunity to learn to take advantage of the many opportunities that are available to everyone who reaches out to accept the positive beginning.

Laura: I know how hard it may seem for someone to adopt this way of life because it's out of the ordinary. I stress, though, that it can be done. Macrobiotics works, if one has the desire to try.

Mrs. Fitzpatrick: As a family macrobiotics brought us much closer, because we all had one center of mutual interest in helping Laura to become well. We found unity and strength in sharing this important aspect of life.

Laura: Moreover, I feel that I am well on my way to a full and complete recovery.

Endometriosis, Tumor in the Colon

Tonia Gagne, Jamaica Plain, Massachusetts, 1981

When I was eighteen, I left home to go to college and became pregnant in my junior year. At this time I started on a health food diet. However, soon after the baby was born, I developed endometriosis, a condition in which the womb and ovaries become infected, and the lining protects itself by growing. If this continues unchecked, the lining starts to warp the internal parts of the womb and ovaries.

Within a year after the baby's birth, I moved into my sister's home. I began to have a profuse vaginal discharge, and was put into the hospital for two months of observation, but my situation did not improve. One day at work I fainted and experienced excruciating pain. Within a week I underwent an operation to remove an ovary and a Fallopian tube. I was put on hormonal therapy (a pill called Enovid 10). The pills were about the size of a dime, and I had to take three every day for nine months. My hair went straight and began to fall out, and my mental state became much worse.

I moved to Boston in 1975 and experienced intermittent pain. Finally, the pain became so bad that I went to a gynecologist in Dorchester who confirmed the endometriosis and also diagnosed a cyst. He told me that the cyst was the size of a small tennis ball. At that point I decided to get more serious about my diet, and so I moved into a macrobiotic study house.

The gynecologist had told me that I would need surgery including a complete hysterectomy. However, the cyst disappeared within three months of eating at the study house, since the cooking there was very simple and I kept myself from binging.

At that time I met my future husband who convinced me to meet with Michio Kushi. Michio could tell simply by looking at me that my left ovary had been removed and that the remaining one was still very diseased. He also said that I had a tumor growing in my descending colon and that I had jaundice. I was very inspired and convinced to follow the diet he recommended.

For the next year I ate very simply. Mentally, I was much improved over what I had been feeling during the past five years. I became very meticulous about housecleaning, went to cooking classes and insisted that everything had to be in perfect order. Anytime I cheated and ate something a little out of line, I would automatically feel severe internal pain. As long as I continued with external treatments and the recommended diet, the pain would be nonexistant.

One day I discharged a lump of cancerous tissue with my bowel movement, and I began to feel much lighter as my intestines also improved.

Within the year, I decided to have a baby, and within a very short time became pregnant. The pregnancy was very easy and comfortable, and I felt no desire to eat animal food. I was quite amazed that this was possible for me. The labor was only four hours long, and Taran was a strong, healthy boy.

I know that I have been very, very arrogant and very sick. Now I find myself much happier and more fulfilled. Macrobiotics isn't any kind of religion or belief system. I had thought that macrobiotics would take the fun out of my life, but instead, I have learned to have more fun. I've learned balance; my life (and sense of enjoyment) is much simpler and much more fulfilling than I have ever before felt.

It's my sincere hope that many, many people will come to the macrobiotic way of life whether they are sick or not. The future lies with our children, and by eating macrobiotically and giving simple values and a simple way of life to those who follow us, we can produce strong, healthy children both in mind and in body. This will ensure a strong, healthy future for out planet.

(In January, 1981, Tonia Gagne gave birth to a second child by natural childbirth at home with no complications, despite an earlier prognosis that she would be unable to have children.)

The Legacy of Jean Kohler

*The following article, written by Tom Monte, is reprinted from
the March, 1981* East West Journal.

Seven and a half years ago, doctors at Indiana University Medical Center told Jean Kohler, a professor of piano at Ball State University in Muncie, Indiana, that he had only a few months to live. The surgeons had found a malignant tumor the size of a fist on Kohler's pancreas as well as infiltration of cancer in his small intestine. They told Kohler that pancreatic cancer was incurable and that he would soon be dead.

After a single dosage of chemotherapy (he took no other medication), Kohler took up the macrobiotic diet. Within a year, medical tests remarkably revealed no signs of cancer. For the next seven years, Kohler wrote letters to scientists, published a book, and gave hundreds of speeches describing his victory over "incurable cancer" through the use of the macrobiotic diet, a regimen made up principally of whole grains and vegetables. Though he maintained that the diet had cured him of cancer and the fact that he was still alive was proof of it, Kohler admitted that the final proof of his victory over this dread disease would not come until he died and his body was autopsied.

On September 14, 1980, Jean Kohler, 63, died in Beth Israel Hospital in Boston of a liver infection and complications resulting from hemorrhaging. According to Beth Israel surgeon Dr. Michael Sobel, Kohler's death "had nothing to do with cancer." Dr. Sobel based this finding on two major exploratory operations which he performed, along with autopsy results and numerous tests and x-rays.

"For someone to survive seven years with cancer of the pancreas without being treated is extremely rare, if not unheard of," Dr. Sobel said. "Something was controlling the cancer."

Kohler's death took friends and colleagues at Ball State—where he was a professor of piano for thirty-three years—completely by surprise. "I was shocked," said Dr. Robert Hargraeves, chairman of the music department at Ball State and a friend of Kohler's since the 1930s when both were graduate students at the Eastman School of Music in Pittsburgh, Pennsylvania. "He was my friend and a truly gifted musician and teacher."

"Jean Kohler was a selfless person whose greatest dream was to spread macrobiotics," said John David Mann, former vice president of the East West Foundation, the macrobiotic educational organization.

Kohler's healing odyssey began in early autumn of 1973, shortly after the doctors gave him up for dead. At that time a friend told him about the macrobiotic diet, which reputedly could cure cancer or extend the patient's life as well as dramatically improve the quality of life during the time remaining. A month later, Jean Kohler and his wife Mary Alice traveled to Boston for a consultation with Michio Kushi, president of the East West Foundation, whose lectures on the nutritional approach to cancer have been attended by doctors and medical students around the world.

After the meeting with Kushi, the Kohlers decided to return to their home in Muncie and begin macrobiotics. They had already been eating their meals several times a week at the home of their friend Mari Samuelson, a gourmet cook. Samuelson was the first of the Kohlers' friends to try the new diet. Many more would follow.

Before beginning macrobiotics, Kohler's illness forced him to sharply cut back his work load at Ball State. However, within a few weeks after beginning the diet, Kohler's strength quickly returned, so much so that he resumed teaching and began an exercise program. For the next eight months, Kohler's condition gradually improved. In April, 1974, blood tests and another consultation with Michio Kushi revealed that all signs of Kohler's cancer were gone.

More than 400,000 Americans die of cancer each year, and after his own successful recovery Kohler was determined to do everything he could to reduce or eliminate those deaths. He wrote hundreds, perhaps thousands, of letters, published a newsletter, wrote articles, made hundreds of speaking engagements, and wrote a book, *Healing Miracles from Macrobiotics* (Parker Publishing Co., 1979). He submitted dozens of articles to major publications, including the *Reader's Digest*, describing his recovery. These efforts failed to bear fruit, however, and Kohler was often frustrated by the fact that millions of people were not beating down his door for the information he was so desperately attempting to spread.

"The validity of the macrobiotic way in helping sick people seemed so obvious to me," he wrote in *Healing Miracles*, and yet so many people, both well and sick, remained unimpressed, that it became an obsession with me to look for ways to spread the news."

It wasn't long before the enthusiastic Jean Kohler joined forces with the East West Foundation. "Many of the programs the Foundation came up with," recalled Ed Esko, former vice president of the Foundation, "were created just so we could provide a forum for Jean Kohler to speak."

Kohler became a featured speaker at such Foundation projects as the annual Amherst Program at Amherst College, Massachusetts, the Cancer Conferences given regularly in Boston, and the 1978 World Without Cancer Conference where Jean Kohler was joined at the podium by author Bill Dufty and film star Gloria Swanson. Kohler also inspired the Foundation to collect case histories, his own among them, and publish them in book form, which the Foundation has done over the years, culminating in the book *Cancer and Diet*.

He dreamed of being on one of the major talk shows and kept a steady stream of mail going out to Merv Griffin, Johnny Carson, and Phil Donahue, explaining his story. He finally got the chance in late 1979 when Philadelphia's PM Magazine show, a local variety program, did a feature that focused on Kohler's dramatic cure and on macrobiotics. The show was subsequently syndicated nationally, once in February, 1980, and again in August of that year.

Like his book and public appearances, the television shows generated hundreds of letters requesting more information about macrobiotics. This should not have been surprising, for Kohler was an articulate speaker whose personality transmitted competence and sincerity. Indeed, Kohler was the kind of man who, upon meeting him, made you feel that you had known him all your life. He was a highly charged man who had that Midwesterner's ability to come right to the point. His face often held a seemingly elfish expression and he appeared to be bubbling over with spirit. All of this combined to make Kohler instantly engaging, so that even if a person didn't believe what he had said, they came away liking him nonetheless.

In March, 1980, a month after the PM Magazine show was aired nationally for the first time, Kohler became ill. At first he said it was just the flu; however, he never fully recovered his strength.

Ironically, the liver infection that was beginning to overtake Kohler and that finally brought about his death may well have been caused by surgery performed in 1973, which found the original tumor growing on his pancreas, Dr. Sobel later speculated. It is hard to say why, after all these years, the infection suddenly became strong enough to bring about such a marked change in Kohler's condition, which had been stable up until last spring. Dr. Sobel said that such infections are often indolent, or very slow-growing. Mary Alice said that her husband had sharply altered his diet in March to combat the effects of the flu. She suggested that this change in diet may have had something to do with Jean's rapid decline.

He was scheduled to speak at the East West Foundation's Amherst Program in August last year, so he and Mary Alice made the trip east to western Massachusetts. Still suffering from the effects of the flu, he was weakened further by the trip. Nevertheless, on August 21, 1980—exactly seven years after exploratory surgery at Indiana revealed a malignant tumor—Kohler spoke before an audience of about 500 people at Amherst and told his story once again.

The following night, he and John David Mann gave a recital for the Amherst Audience—Kohler on piano and Mann on cello. They played a Beethoven sonata and it was clear then that Kohler's illness was quickly overtaking him. "He was barely able to keep up with the piece," said Mann.

After the conclusion of the Amherst Program, Michio Kushi advised Kohler to take some time off and stay at the Manns' home. Kohler spent about a week at the Manns', until August 30, when it was apparent that the best place for him was Beth Israel Hospital. By then the liver infection had caused Kohler's stomach to swell considerably, and he was in tremendous pain.

"In all that ensued we were swept along by destiny," Mary Alice wrote in an open letter to friends. "During the previous seven years it always seemed, as we kept saying, that things consistently fell into place in our favor. But now it seemed as if one piece of bad luck catapulted us toward another."

Kohler spent the night in the emergency ward at Beth Israel, the pain keeping him from sleep.

Michio Kushi, along with several other friends of Kohler's including a macrobiotic medical doctor, joined him in his room. They all conferred with Dr. Sobel and other Beth Israel physicians. The Beth Israel doctors advised Kohler to submit to surgery. The physicians believed that Kohler was once again beset by cancer. "No one gets over pancreatic cancer," Mary Alice remembers one physician saying.

"Since he was still mentally alert the choice was his," Mary Alice said. "So I asked him whether we should wait. He shook his head. Hoping I misunderstood, I asked, 'Do you mean you want the surgery?' I had to put my ear very close to his lips to hear his whisper."

" 'I'm too weak to explain,' Jean said, 'but I have to do this.' "

Dr. Sobel performed the operation and drained the abscess on Kohler's liver and a great deal of infection from his intestines. He then told Mary Alice that there had been no sign of cancer.

One more major surgery and two minor ones failed to rescue Kohler from the liver infection and the massive amount of hemorrhaging that was taking place in his intestines.

On September 14 he died.

Any doubts that Kohler had indeed survived an "incurable cancer" were quickly put to rest with the ensuing autopsy. The results provided some startling revelations. According to Dr. Sobel, "microscopic cancer cells" were found in Kohler's pancreas. However, Dr. Sobel concluded, "What we can say about Jean Kohler's case is that over the past seven years his cancer had actually gotten smaller. He started out having a large tumor in the pancreas and seven years later the cancer was microscopic." Dr. Sobel pointed out that Kohler was "in no immediate danger from the cancer" and that the cancer cells found were in no way related to his death.

Thus, over the past seven years, Kohler's body was healing itself; his once virulent cancer ultimately became little more than microscopic cells that provided no immediate danger.

In submitting to the surgery at Beth Israel, coupled with the results of the autopsy, Kohler provided the strongest evidence yet that he had survived an incurable cancer, which had been controlled by no other means than his body's own natural defenses. He maintained throughout the past seven years that those defenses were made capable of staving off the cancer and, indeed, shrinking the tumor, because of his adherence to a balanced diet of whole grains and vegetables.

Thus, even in death, Kohler continued to give to others what he had given in life—hope and faith in our ability to defeat disease by harmonizing with the order of nature.

Meanwhile, Mary Alice still hears Jean's whisper, "I'm too weak to explain, but I have to do this."

John Jodziewicz:
A Young Man's Journey Back to Life

*The following article, written by Tom Monte, is reprinted from
the April, 1982* East West Journal.

On March 23, 1980, John Jodziewicz then 23 years old, sat in a hospital bed and contemplated his own imminent death. He and his fiancee, Ingrid Koch, had just heard the diagnosis from his physicians: pure choriocarcinoma, stage IV, of the left testicle, which had metastacized to both lungs, the left kidney, and neck. His physicians had given him a two percent chance of living out the year. After his doctors had left them alone, John and Ingrid sat on his bed and held on to one another like two people caught in a hurricane. Both were determined that John was not going to die.

Today, John Jodziewicz (pronounced Ujevitz) sits before me and talks about the future as if it were a banquet he was about to devour. His hair, which had all fallen out due to several months of chemotherapy in 1980, is now almost entirely grown back. At five feet nine inches and 150 pounds he is trim and fit, and there are times when he looks, for all the world, like a Polish Omar Sharif. In May, 1981, blood tests revealed that there was no sign of cancer left in his body. The final proof that he is completely free of cancer will have to wait until John feels ready for chest x-rays. But he's not in any hurry. John says he's got many years ahead of him to prove he has conquered his disease.

What follows is the story of one man's struggle against cancer. It is not merely the story of a successful application of technology, or even diet, though both played vital roles in John Jodziewicz's miraculous recovery. It is more the story of one man's refusal to be defeated and the role spiritual consciousness plays in the fight everyone wages against adversity, whether it be against a dread disease such as cancer, or the apparently insurmountable challenges that life places before us.

It was the summer of 1977 that John first noticed a pea-shaped growth on his left testicle. The growth immediately worried him, but he rationalized the fear away; it's a small infection that will pass, he told himself.

He was a sophomore at Kutztown State College, in Kutztown, Pennsylvania. Two years later, he graduated and had plans to attend graduate school and study geology, once he had saved enough money for tuition and expenses.

But in the early part of 1980, the growth had caused his testicle to become swollen and painful. Also, a lump had developed at the base of his neck, just above the collarbone. It hadn't occurred to John that the two symptoms might be connected, but the testicle worried him. He decided it was time to see an endocrinologist in his hometown of Allentown, Pennsylvania.

When the physician examined John's testicle and the lump on his neck, he immediately became alarmed.

"Stay here, I have to make a telephone call," he told John. With that he rushed into his outer office and called another doctor. Now more afraid than ever, John pressed his ear against the wall in an effort to hear the doctor's conversation—but to no avail. In a few moments, the doctor rushed back into his inner office and handed John a slip of paper with the name and address of another doctor who would see John immediately.

"What's the problem?" John asked. The doctor looked at John for an instant and then said, "It's malignant."

"From that point on," John recalls, "everything moved fast. There was a sense of urgency about every move my doctors made." John would quickly find out that his doctors did not believe there was a moment to lose in their efforts to save his life.

John was sent to an oncologist, a doctor who specializes in the diagnosis and treatment of cancer. The doctor examined John and immediately ordered him to enter Allentown Sacred Heart Hospital, where he scheduled a radical left orchiectomy, which is the surgical removal of the left testicle.

John entered Sacred Heart Hospital on March 19, 1980, underwent a battery of tests, including x-rays, and was operated on the following day. His left testicle was removed and then analyzed for cancer. For the next three days, John and Ingrid waited in his room for the results of the biopsy. John was still reeling from the trauma of losing a testicle. Although he would still be capable of procreation, the psychological impact of the operation left him emotionally shaken. On the third day, he and Ingrid were sitting in his room when suddenly a nurse came into the room and in a very business-like manner pulled closed a curtain that hung from the ceiling between John's bed and his roommate. The nurse then left them without a word. In a few moments, three doctors entered John's room with bad news written all over their faces.

They explained to John that the testicle had been biopsied several times and the results were conclusive: pure choriocarcinoma of the testicle, which is a type of cancer of the testicle that does not respond well to treatment. The cancer had spread to his left kidney, both lungs, and his neck. As soon as he had recovered from surgery, the doctors planned to implement chemotherapy, which is essentially administration of a drug toxic to cancer cells—and other body cells, as well—in an effort to destroy the cancer.

Still, when John heard the word therapy, he immediately felt some small hope. Images of physical therapy and of wonder drugs came to his mind. John didn't know what chemotherapy was. These hopeful thoughts were quickly dampened, however.

"John, I hope you realize the severity of the situation," one doctor told him. Suddenly, John was aware that the three doctors were waiting for him to react; they stood poised and silent. Then he felt the impact of what was being said.

"I guess you're all waiting for the denial stage," John said, in a reference to Elizabeth Kubler Ross's *Death and Dying*, in which Ross outlines the stages a person goes through in the process of coming to grips with one's own death.

No one answered John's comment. "What are my chances of living?" he asked. He was then informed that his chances were extremely poor—perhaps a two percent chance that he would survive the year. Shortly thereafter, the doctors left John and Ingrid alone. For some reason, John was keenly aware that none of the doctors had physically touched him.

Gradually, the shock crept in on him, like the slow effects of an anesthetic. Soon he was numb.

"How do you react to news like that?" he asks today. "It's like walking up to the Grand Canyon and seeing it for the first time. What can you say about it?"

A day or two after John received the news, a young intern came into his room.

97

He sat on John's bed and the two talked for a time. John felt comforted. Toward the end of their conversation, the doctor placed his hand on John's knee and looked at him hard. "John, have you ever considered an alternative?" he said. The word "laetrile" lit up in John's mind. John realized that the young physician was treading on dangerous ground, so he didn't press matters; the point was made. With that the intern left him. Later, when John inquired of the doctor's whereabouts, he was informed that he had been transferred to another hospital.

The thought of an alternative had already crossed Ingrid's mind. Ingrid is an attractive woman with long brown hair, hazel eyes, and a heart-shaped face. She was born and raised in northeast Philadelphia and at thirteen her parents divorced. From that point on, she assumed much of the responsibility for the care of her younger brother while her mother worked. Like many children who have responsibility thrust on them at a young age, Ingrid grew up strong and skeptical of everything, particularly of powerful institutions such as medicine and organized religion.

After she graduated from high school, Ingrid attended Kutztown State College, where she met John, and graduated with a degree in psychology. She then took a job working with mentally retarded adults. Now, in order to devote more time to John, she had all her hours shifted to the weekend and spent the rest of the week in the hospital where John was recovering from surgery and would soon begin chemotherapy. At the same time, she began making calls all over the country about laetrile, or any other type of alternative cancer therapy that people would talk about. Nothing seemed to hold out much hope, however. In fact, the more she found out about the alternative treatments, including laetrile, the more disheartened she became. At the same time, Ingrid began to investigate the likelihood that chemotherapy would save John's life. The chances of that happening, she soon found out, were also painfully slim.

John also started to poke around for alternatives to chemotherapy. One day he asked his own chief physician, the man who would supervise John's treatment, whether he had examined the alternatives with an open mind. The doctor said he had. "Everyone who followed an alternative cancer approach is dead now," John recalls his doctor saying. John pressed the issue. John told the doctor that another physician treating him had given him only a two percent chance of living out the year; in light of such poor prognosis, wouldn't it be better if John simply abstained from all drugs?

"Everyone has a 50/50 chance of making it," the doctor stated angrily. "Everyone!" At that point, John agreed to go ahead with the chemotherapy.

The chemotherapy was scheduled to begin on March 26. The night before, John walked up and down the halls of the ward. In a room well down the hall from his own, John heard the wretching and vomiting of an old woman. The woman was in such a tortured state that it seemed she might succumb from the vomiting. "What's wrong with that woman?" John asked a nurse on the ward. The old woman was getting chemotherapy, the nurse said.

"Does everyone get sick like that?" John asked.

"Not everyone," was the nurse's reply. The optimistic sound of the word therapy evaporated in John's mind like a droplet in the desert.

The next morning John was given a paper to read that listed the side-effects of chemotherapy. These included vomiting, bleeding, loss of white blood cells, and bone marrow depression. There would be pain in the bones and joints and he might bruise easily.

That morning John had made the mistake of eating a heavy breakfast of potato pancakes. A short time after breakfast, a nurse and physician wheeled into John's room a cart containing drugs, including chemotherapy, and intravenous equipment. The chemotherapy and other drugs were contained in bottles that were suspended from a stand, which John referred to as "the tree." Chemotherapy was given intravenously over seven days.

John hated needles, especially cold ones. While his physician probed John's arm searching for a good vein to insert the intravenous needle into, John closed his eyes and pressed his forefinger and thumb together until they nearly crushed each other. Finally, the cold steel broke the skin and found a vein. Sugar water and then compazine—a drug used to reduce vomiting—flowed into his veins. Then came the chemotherapy.

Shortly thereafter, the vomiting started.

"I vomited so much that there was nothing left to bring up but bile," John said recently. "I couldn't go near potato pancakes for months."

John is not the type of person who likes to impose on others, and now, as he violently and noisily convulsed, he kept thinking of how he must be affecting his roommate. John apologized profusely but realized that this only made his roommate more uncomfortable. John kept thinking of the old woman and how someone should have shut her away, so he got into the habit of bringing his chemotherapy cart, his "tree," into the bathroom, where he could turn on the shower and the faucet and keep the toilet flushing. He drowned himself out and, somehow, the sound of rushing water made things more bearable.

John was on a typical chemotherapy routine of seven days continuous treatment. At the conclusion of the seven days, he was allowed to go home and recuperate. At this point, he was very vulnerable to disease. Chemotherapy wipes out white blood cells, thus destroying the body's resistance. John's doctors were particularly concerned that he would contract pneumonia. Because hospitals are places where bacteria run rampant, it was better for him to go home to recover. When the white blood cell count returned to normal—usually within two or three weeks—John would return to the hospital to undergo another seven days of continuous chemotherapy.

During the first seven days in the hospital, John spent a lot of time in the bathroom listening to the water run. Because chemotherapy is essentially toxic to the system, the doctors kept a close watch on how much of the drug went into John's body and how much liquid he expelled through the urine and vomit. If the chemotherapy wasn't adequately discharged, it would have an extremely debilitating effect on the kidneys and lungs. Drugs are usually administered to help the kidneys flush out the chemotherapy, if they aren't already doing this on their own.

On top of the vomiting, John's skin itched profusely from the compazine. "There were times when I just wanted to jump out of my skin," John recalls.

Ingrid tried to comfort him. She would wash his face, try to get him to eat, and do everything possible to lift his spirits. She filled his room with plants and flowers.

Meanwhile, the hospital staff made use of her by having her measure the liquid John expelled, making sure he maintained a certain level that would indicate the chemotherapy was being discharged from his system.

"John was beside himself," Ingrid said recently. "I was afraid he was starting to lose touch with reality."

John's mother had been dead for seven years, but his father and stepmother visited him regularly. Ingrid was with him all day until visiting hours ended at 8 p.m. There were times, however, when he would drift inside himself and no one would be able to reach him.

John always loved rainy days; he thought they were special for him. When he was in the hospital it seemed to rain a lot. Some days he would press his face up against the window and look out at the wet, green Pennsylvania countryside, as the rain made long tears against the windowpane.

"If the window hadn't been locked, I might have jumped," said John.

After a few days on chemotherapy, John became acquainted with some other young men who also had cancer and were being treated with chemotherapy. They too were suffering from the toxic effects of the treatments, but they had help getting through the day: They were all smoking marijuana. Everyday, they would gather in one of the bathrooms and "toke up." One day, one of the members of this little fraternity offered John a marijuana cigarette. At first, John resisted. He had never taken drugs in his life. When he was a senior in college, he became a vegetarian and considered himself a health-nut. He took vitamins and supplements and ate a vegetarian diet of mostly dairy foods, bread, and sweets. Now, as the young man offered him the marijuana, John resisted, thinking perhaps that it was no good for his health, but of course that was a ludicrous thought. He was dying of cancer; he needed something to help him keep his sanity, so he took the joint and joined the others in the bathroom each day. The marijuana seemed to calm his system and reduce the vomiting.

At the end of the first week, John went home to Henningsville, Pennsylvania, which is outside of Allentown. John thought it might be better at home, but it wasn't. He developed enormous mouth sores and nose bleeds; his whole body became arthritic, with terrible pain in his head and joints. All his hair fell out, and his beard shed like an old dog in the summer. His weight dropped from around 210 to 170 in a matter of weeks. The vomiting continued, and he found it impossible to eat. Soon, he found his teeth were coming loose. He couldn't seem to get comfortable, no matter how he would sit or lay. Ingrid tried giving him a soft massage, but his skin felt like it was being electrocuted. At night he would curl up in the fetal position and fall into a shallow and fitful sleep.

Marijuana became more precious to him than gold.

After about two weeks at home, the mouth sores would pass and his appetite would return. However, that usually indicated that his white blood cell count had returned to normal and it was time to return to the hospital.

The second week in the hospital was like the first. During the day, the little group of cancer patients would gather in the bathroom, each of them attached to their "trees" by the intravenous lines that were strung from them like umbilical cords. They were all as bald as babies—usually balder. They passed around the marijuana like a secret password among prisoners. Everyone was pulling for one another. They were afraid that if any one member of the group died, they would all follow in rapid succession.

One of the members of the group was named Speed. Speed's girlfriend used to come to John secretly and give him pep talks about how he had to survive. "If you don't make it, John, then Speed's not going to make it."

"It was like 'Stalag 17' or 'One Flew Over the Cuckoo's Nest,' " said John. They had this awful thing in common and they held onto it like precious life. Each night, the group would meet in John's room and watch MASH. After MASH, visiting hours were over and everyone would scatter. Ingrid would have to leave and John would go down to the chapel alone.

John was brought up a strict Roman Catholic and a proud Polish-American. He likes to remind people that there are more than sixty towns and cities in the United States named after Polish cities; that Polish General Thaddeus Kosciuszko was an American Revolutionary War hero; and that Solidarity will never die. Like the Polish people themselves, John's link to the mother church is both sustenance for the soul and the very symbol of a Pole's refusal to give up the fight against oppression. In some ways, John saw his disease as yet another invader of Polish territory that had to be fought off. He prayed that God would not allow his will and strength to be broken. However, if it was God's will that he die, John wanted to be prepared. After an hour or so in the chapel, John would wheel his "tree" back into his room and sleep a little more easily.

His doctors were constantly checking the effects the chemotherapy was having on the tumors. Almost every other day, John was being x-rayed in order to determine how the cancer was reacting to the treatment. No one was giving him good news.

After the second trip to the hospital was over, John returned home for three more weeks. The mouth sores became so bad that it was as if he had been chewing on razor blades. In truth, he couldn't chew anything; he had no appetite, nor could he keep anything down. He decided to fast—or perhaps there was no alternative but to fast. Meanwhile, Ingrid did what little she could to make him comfortable. John would say later that at this point it seemed as if both of them had cancer.

When John came back to the hospital for the third time, his doctors had decided that the regular dosages of chemotherapy were not working. They explained that his case was very severe and that extraordinary measures were necessary. They had checked with researchers at the University of Indiana Medical School who had recommended the use of experimental dosages of a new drug called sis platinum in combination with the chemotherapy routine. Because the sis platinum was so powerful and had numerous side-effects, they would shorten the protocol from seven to five days. His doctors asked John if he knew anyone who could donate blood in case he needed a large transfusion. He gave them his sister's name.

Later John was visited by a single doctor who told him more specifically what the side-effects of the sis platinum might be. The doctor appeared deeply depressed. He explained that sis platinum would be administered only twice, since it was highly toxic to the system. He intimated to John that there was some danger in the size of the dosage and it could be very harmful and perhaps lethal. In any event, the earlier dosages of chemotherapy were not having the desired results, and this course was thought to be necessary.

At this point, John asked him what specifically would kill him and how would he die? Probably his lungs would go. John was told. However, he shouldn't worry; there were plenty of drugs to keep him from suffering a painful death.

John and Ingrid were terrified. After a while, John called his father and step-mother. John always derived a great deal of strength from his father. "My father is a strong man," he said. "His name is Zygmut Casimire Jodziewicz; the first two names are the names of two kings of Poland—I always liked the sound of my father's name."

He called his father now and told him what was happening. He could not keep back the tears. His father also became choked up. He said he'd come down to the hospital immediately.

That night John, Ingrid, and John's parents sat in his room and watched MASH. After MASH was over, everyone went down to the chapel and prayed hard. There was a lot of soul searching into the night.

The next morning, John's parents and Ingrid were with John when the sis platinum was wheeled into the room on the cart with the tree. Almost ominously, the sis platinum was kept in aluminum foil in order to protect it from the light. It was then administered intravenously, as the chemotherapy had been.

It wasn't long after the drug was circulating through his system that John began to vomit profusely and then lapsed into convulsions. Ingrid and John's stepmother, Anna Jodziewicz, held onto John while he wretched and shook like a man in an electric chair.

The convulsion soon became worse and John could feel himself losing his grip.

"I started to feel as if I could just let go and die right there," he said. "I felt like I could take off right out of my body."

The convulsions continued to rack his body and drive his consciousness into some deep recess of his psyche. Suddenly, John let go. He stopped holding on and just floated to the ceiling of the room. For a moment, he was looking down at his body and saw Ingrid and his stepmother holding him; it looked like a tragi-comedy, he thought. For some reason, he felt a vague sense of guilt; he knew he was putting these people through a lot of pain, and he knew too that it would be a terrible crime to die in their arms. In a moment he was back in his body and his consciousness was returning. He could hear Ingrid's voice.

"Smoke one, John. You've got to smoke one," she was saying.

"No, I can't," he heard himself say.

"John, you've got to smoke one. Now go ahead and take it."

He saw Ingrid offer him a joint. Then he looked at his father. He was utterly ashamed.

"Dad, I'm not a drug addict," John blurted out.

"John, if it makes you feel better, then smoke it," his father said.

John got control of himself. He wanted to go into the bathroom where he could be alone. Ingrid had to help him. John pulled his "tree" into the bathroom, turned on the shower and the faucet, and got stoned.

The day had left him exhausted and that night he fell into a bottomless sleep. With an almost terrifying clarity, he dreamt of his mother. It was just a short dream; she simply came before him and told him, "John, go to St. Joseph's."

John knew what his mother meant. Many years before, when John was still a child, his parents took him to St. Joseph's Cathedral in Montreal, Canada. St. Joseph's Cathedral is the place where Father Alfred Bessette, better known throughout Canada as Brother André, reportedly performed many miracles, including healing the sick. Today, thousands of pilgrims from all over the world travel to

St. Joseph's to go up the many steps on their knees to the top of the mountain. This show of humility and reverence is made in hopes that God will bless them and heal their illness.

As a child, John was very impressed with the sight of so many people going up the mountain steps on their knees. He was also moved by the sight of the many sets of crutches and canes that were left behind in the cathedral by the sick who came away well after going up the steps, either on their own power or with the help of others.

Now, John's dream made clear to him what he had to do: He must go to St. Joseph's and go up the steps on his knees.

By the end of the week, he was discharged from the hospital and he spent the next three weeks recuperating. At that time, Ingrid's mother, who had been sick with lupus disease, was practicing macrobiotics. Her friend, Kurt Maunte, had introduced Ingrid's mother to macrobiotics after reading about the diet and philosophy in a magazine. Now, Kurt Maunte urged John to meet Denny Waxman, director of the Philadelphia East West Foundation and a long-time student of marcobiotics. On a whim, John went along.

Waxman gave John a consultation and then told him of the standard macrobiotic diet, which Waxman said could help John get well. Waxman outlined the diet John should follow as approximately 60 percent whole grains and about 30 percent locally grown vegetables, and the rest beans, sea vegetables, certain soups, and condiments. John looked at the recommendations Waxman had listed on a piece of paper, and told Waxman he'd think it over. After he left Waxman, John bought two books—*The Book of Macrobiotics* and *The Book of Do-In*, both by Michio Kushi, the macrobiotic educator.

Ingrid and John read the books and considered going on the diet. Meanwhile, John's three weeks of recuperation were over and he went back into the hospital for another five days of sis platinum and chemotherapy. Again John suffered vomiting and tremors, though he did not experience the intense convulsions that he had experienced the first time he took the sis platinum. He continued to smoke marijuana heavily.

The mental image of his mother seemed to be always with him now.

After the second round of sis platinum was concluded, John underwent another battery of tests. X-rays revealed that the tumors in his lungs were still present; the right tumor was as large as ever, but the left showed some shrinkage. The tumor in his neck had not changed. On the other hand, John's blood tests had improved markedly and were now virtually normal. Still, it was hoped that the sis platinum would eradicate the tumors or accomplish more toward reducing them in size. The fact that they were still present was not a good sign.

Just before he left the hospital, John asked one of his physicians how much time he might have left before the tumor in his lung killed him. The answer he got was perhaps a couple of months.

Now it was the end of May and John felt sick in body and soul; he had no energy and seemed constantly lethargic; his teeth were loose; the mouth sores were back; he had no appetite; he couldn't walk for any distance before he had to rest. The vomiting continued. He felt as if he was existing in some nether world between life and death.

Ingrid could see clearly that John was on the ropes. She told him that she

103

didn't think chemotherapy was accomplishing anything. It was obvious to her that the chemotherapy was killing John faster than the cancer. "What do you want to die of, John?" she finally asked him. John knew he didn't want to die in the hospital. Together they looked over the recommendations Waxman had given him. They also read the books. Finally, they decided to begin macrobiotics. At this point, John stopped all medication, including chemotherapy, and did not resume it.

Although she encouraged him to follow macrobiotics, Ingrid's ever-present skepticism prevented her from thinking that the diet was going to provide John with anything more than hope for the future. Still, in the state he was in, even that was a lot to ask for, Ingrid said recently.

After they had decided to begin macrobiotics, John told Ingrid of his plan to go to Montreal and climb the steps of St. Joseph's. Ingrid was more incredulous of the steps than she was of macrobiotics, but she told him she would go along.

"My feeling was that if John wants to go and crawl up those steps then that's what he's got to do," Ingrid said later. "I figured it was the psychological part of what he had to do to cure himself." Nevertheless, as the two of them drove to Montreal in John's Volkswagen bus in the middle of June, Ingrid thought more than once that "If John lives, I'll believe in God." Such thoughts she kept to herself, however. She knew she was one of the tenuous threads from which his life hung.

They arrived in Montreal on June 16, St. John Baptiste Day, a day that was as perfect as a spring flower. St. Joseph's Cathedral seemed to bask in the sun atop its high mountain where it overlooked the entire city.

The city was in celebration and tourists were everywhere. When John and Ingrid drove up to the foot of the mountain, both of them suddenly panicked. There were no pilgrims going up the steps. There were only tourists walking around the grounds, all dressed up in their short sleeve shirts and wearing cameras around their necks as if this was some international convention of paparazzi. There was a lot of high-pitched laughter, roaming eyes, and the idle chatter of people with nothing but time on their hands. The center aisle of steps, which is reserved for the faithful, was empty. Suddenly, St. Joseph's appeared to be more an historical monument than a place of miracles.

"Am I going to go up those steps on my knees and humiliate myself in front of thousands of tourists?" John asked himself. For a moment he was overwhelmed by the urge to turn back. He looked at the mountain again and remembered his dream.

"Ingrid, don't look," John said.

"Don't worry, John, I can't," Ingrid told him.

John went to the foot of the mountain and the bottom step. Ingrid went for a walk.

To the many tourists who saw John walk up to the middle aisle and place his knees on the step, he must have looked like a born-again Kojak. He was completely bald and clean-shaven. The careful observer might have seen the large dark rings around his eyes, or his drawn and sallow skin. That observer might have guessed that John had cancer and was now desperately in need of a miracle. But probably no one took careful notice of him. John doesn't remember, because by the time he reached the foot of the mountain he was in a trance.

When he placed his knees on the step, he experienced a transcendent moment. He felt as if he had become part of the very mountain. All the tourists, all the chatter, all the idle time—faded. It was only John The Mountain. He started climbing.

John was taught at a young age that one never prays for oneself. God knows what you need; you don't have to ask. So you pray for others and hope that as God dispenses his blessings, you're among the blessed. John had made a list of his relatives, ancestors, and friends who needed help, and at every step he prayed for someone on the list. As he ascended each step, he felt the presence of his mother's spirit closer and closer. And with every step he took, he felt a growing confidence that all would be well. He would regain his health. He would practice macrobiotics and the tumors would disappear. He would have help from above. His life was about to turn around.

Somewhere near the top a step was covered with a pool of water, probably from a recent rain. John's knees were killing him. When he placed them in the water on the step, the pain vanished and elation flowed through him like the breath of new life. He stayed on that step, kneeling in the water, for a few long moments.

Soon, he got to the top step. He took a deep breath and walked into the cathedral.

He came into the cathedral at the tail end of a Mass, and communion was almost over. John had no intention of taking part in the service; he wanted to go into the chapel where he could light some candles and pray a while longer. But just as he entered the church and looked to the altar, he saw the priest standing there, holding up the wafer. The timing was uncanny; the priest seemed to be waiting for John. John realized that this was his cue. He went to the altar and took communion.

Then he went into the chapel and lit some candles and prayed.

Ingrid joined him in the chapel and together they came down from the mountain.

John and Ingrid toured Montreal, which seemed to them an Emerald City. They both felt as if they had awakened from a long and terrible nightmare.

When John and Ingrid returned to Pennsylvania, they attended the East West Foundation's Mid-Atlantic Summer Camp, which at that time was held in Kintersville, Pennsylvania. There they met Stan and Geraldine Walker, with whom John and Ingrid would begin studying macrobiotics as part of the East West Foundation's education programs.

At the summer camp, John also had a consultation with Michio Kushi. After talking to John about his condition for a time, Kushi told him that he could recover. He would have to eat a strict macrobiotic diet. However, Kushi said that he could have a little fruit—perhaps a few raisins—if he really craved it. John would hold strictly to this diet for the next year.

"Every time I craved something sweet, I would put a couple of raisins in my palm and ask myself, 'Do I really need these?' Usually, the answer was no," John said.

Once he began the macrobiotic diet, John's strength returned quickly.

"John's motto is nothing in moderation," said Ingrid. "Once he started the diet and began exercising, he did everything in extremes."

John and Ingrid went to the Walkers' house for cooking classes and meals three or four times a week. When Ingrid couldn't make it, John would often ride his bicycle from Henningsville to Philadelphia, some seventy-five miles away.

When she first started macrobiotics, Ingrid was highly skeptical of the substance of the diet and philosophy. She hoped it would help John psychologically, which might in turn help him with his cancer. More than that she wouldn't ask for. But as the weeks went by, she saw the food was having a powerful effect on both of them. "I could see the diet was working," Ingrid said. "Everything Denny or the Walkers said would happen to him happened. When they told me to give him a certain food for a recurring symptom it always worked. I was real skeptical in the beginning, but I could see it was doing him a lot of good. It even was helping me feel better."

By the end of the summer of 1980, John was feeling pretty much like a bull moose. He had always loved hiking and he loved the Appalachian Trail. There was a thirty-eight-mile stretch of it that he had always wanted to hike and he thought that now was the time to do it. Against Ingrid's advice, John set out on his thirty-eight-mile jaunt. He told Ingrid to meet him at the end of the trail the following day. He took his dog along for company.

"The next day, I met John at the end of the trail," Ingrid said. "The dog was exhausted but John was feeling fine and chipper. I had to help the dog get into the car, while John was cracking jokes. He always amazed me with his strength before the cancer, and I knew then that he was pretty much back to normal." Everyday, John went to the gym to work out. Even he couldn't believe how good he was feeling after so short a time.

"I started to feel better after a week on the diet," he said. "Right away, I had more vitality and I just felt happier and stronger. I just had a very positive attitude right from the start."

"I never really thought he'd die," said Ingrid. "I tried to picture him dying and I just couldn't. I always saw him alive."

In May, 1981, John had a second blood test which showed there was still no sign of cancer. He had been off all medication, including chemotherapy, for a year. Meanwhile, his strength improved by quantum leaps and the tumor in his neck virtually disappeared. He says he feels better today than he did when he was a high school football player. Moreover, this improvement has come in the face of his physician's prognosis that he would probably not survive 1980. Frequent attempts to contact his doctors for a statement or comment on John's recovery have all proven futile; however, John is in custody of all his medical records and is happy to share them with interested medical professionals.

John plans to have chest x-rays, perhaps the final proof that he is well, sometime within the next year. Nevertheless, with or without the x-rays, no one could convince him that he is in anything but a state of wellness.

Today, John is studying macrobiotics at the Kushi Institute in Boston. He hopes eventually to use macrobiotics as a basis for helping others to make changes in their spiritual paths, their lifestyles, and their health.

At this point, one might ask: "What is the cause of John Jodziewicz's recovery?" Some will say it is the chemotherapy, although he was on chemotherapy only four months, and the prognosis even with it was poor at best. Someone else might point to John's spiritual attitude and say it was a miracle, or to Ingrid's support and say it was the power of love. Others will say it was John's healing diet that brought about his recovery. Still others will argue that John's cancer is simply in remission, and thus a temporary phenomenon.

There is still another point of view, which posits that all of these factors together resulted in the remission of John's cancer. All the treatment, all the love, his healing diet, and his basic reverence for life and for God all combined to bring about his improved health. Chemotherapy, diet, and Ingrid's loving support might have failed if used individually. Indeed, we have seen each of these methods fail too many times already. But all of them taken together, coupled with John's awareness of some higher, more powerful spiritual presence, may well have been his ticket out of death and into a new life. This is what makes John's case hopeful and worthy of study. For if one person can blaze the trail and show us the way, then others can surely follow.

Tonia's Triumph Over Illness and Infertility

The following article, written by Tom Monte, is reprinted from
the March, 1982 East West Journal.

It is a classical domestic scene. Two children are playing on the living room floor. Taran, a boy of three, plays absent-mindedly with a toy pistol while his one-year-old sister, Shayla, waddles across the room toward the window where the morning sun pours in and splashes on the living room floor. Tonia Gagne, thirty-two, runs after her daughter and finally nabs her. Gently, she lays Shayla down on the floor and finishes dressing her.

Tonia makes a joke about mother's work never being done while she fits a second pin into Shayla's diaper. Meanwhile, Taran decides he wants to go outside; when his mother says he'll have to wait, Taran begins to cry and stomp about. As compensation, Tonia hands Taran a rice cake and he seems momentarily satisfied. In five minutes, however, Tonia will have to break up a brawl between Taran and Shayla over the rice cakes, and during the next hour she will have to patiently stop what she is doing every few minutes to answer the demands of her children.

It's true: mother's work is never done, but Tonia's smile never withers. Somewhere, not far from her conscious mind, is her doctor's voice telling her that she probably would never have children.

Tonia Gagne is slim, five feet six inches tall, with long curly black hair, large brown eyes behind her glasses, and a ready, energetic smile. She and her husband, Steve, live with their two children in a two-story house in Jamaica Plain, a section of Boston.

Nine years ago, Tonia was diagnosed as having endometriosis, a disease that results from implantation of tissue within the walls of the uterus and around the bowels and the ovaries. This tissue, which is part of the endometrium, should shed and be discharged with the monthly menstrual cycle. However, with endometriosis, part of the tissue remains behind and implants within the pelvis, causing bleeding, pain, irregular and difficult menstrual periods, and often infertility. Today, doctors point out that endometriosis is virtually an epidemic among young and middle-aged women. The standard cure for the disease is to remove the ovaries—and thus the woman's ability to conceive. However, sometimes certain therapies and surgery can halt the spread of the tissue implants. Nevertheless, many women routinely undergo a hysterectomy in order to completely eliminate the problem from their lives.

When her doctors discovered that she had endometriosis, Tonia underwent surgery and had her left ovary removed. As a matter of course, the surgeon also decided to take out her appendix. However, in 1976, her doctors informed her that the endometriosis had not been cured by the original surgery and recommended that she undergo another operation to have the right ovary removed as well. She contemplated having the operation as advised but decided against it. Instead Tonia took up the macrobiotic diet, a regimen composed chiefly of whole grains and vegetables. Within a year after starting the diet, her endometriosis was gone and she conceived her son Taran. Three years later, Tonia conceived her daughter

Shayla. Today, doctors have diagnosed Tonia as having no sign of endometriosis nor the uterine cysts she was diagnosed as having five years ago.

While Tonia relates her story, I watch as she breaks every few moments to answer Taran and Shayla's endless queries. There's a quiet strength in Tonia, the kind that radiates from within and comes only with commitment to a difficult task. This is not a woman who has had it easy; this is a woman who's come to know her priorities through experience. And yet, that wide-open look in her eye, the ever-ready smile, seem to radiate a kind of freshness of youth and innocence.

These are rare qualities in someone who's been over the bumpy road. For Tonia Gagne did not just defeat a so-called incurable disease; she rescued herself from a lifestyle that was pulling her into the grave.

"I'm a person of extremes," Tonia admits. "Inside me is a devil and a nun."

In 1968, Tonia left her parents' home in Long Island, New York, to attend college at the State University of New York, located in St. Pauls, New York. For a young man or woman who has never lived away from their parents, college means more than just education; college often translates into escape and rebellion. In part, Tonia was rebelling against her parents, particularly her mother, a devoted and religious woman who seemed to get little in return for her life of hardship. Tonia wasn't looking for hardship; she was looking for the fast lane.

When she got to college, she immediately found her way into the party life. "I didn't take drugs," she says, "but I liked to drink." After a few semesters at school, Tonia had a steady boyfriend and in January, 1971, she found herself pregnant.

She didn't believe in abortion. "I always believed that life begins at conception," she says. Yet, she was not prepared to raise a child nor marry her boyfriend. The feeling of her boyfriend was mutual. So Tonia carried the child for the full nine months and after she gave birth gave the baby up for adoption.

Giving up a baby she carried for nine months was far more traumatic for Tonia than she could ever have anticipated. Something inside her snapped.

"It broke my heart to give up the child; after that I just went a little crazy," Tonia recalls.

It wasn't long before she began to lose her grip on reality. She started to feel removed from other people. Alienation set in. Fear immobilized her like a straight-jacket.

"I went to a party some friends had given me and somebody poured some wine," she recalls. "I looked down at the wine pouring and suddenly I saw the wine moving really slow; everything was moving in slow motion. Even voices started to become real slow."

Then she had a nervous breakdown.

Soon, her sister asked her to come to Gloversville, New York, where she could minister to Tonia and nurse her back to health. Tonia agreed to go. When she got to Gloversville, however, a deep depression set in and some frightening physical symptoms started to surface. She had hot flashes and cold sweats. Her menstrual cycle went haywire, and she suffered from vaginal discharges and agonizing cramps. She also had headaches and became easily fatigued. She was already under medical care for her mental state and now had to see a gynecologist.

However, just before she saw the gynecologist, she decided to change her diet. Her old boyfriend ate health foods, and he had told her that certain foods were detrimental to the reproductive organs. She didn't know whether he was right or wrong, but she decided she would give up eating meat anyway.

"Something inside me was just beginning to make the connection that food can have a big impact on our health."

Meanwhile, she went to a gynecologist, Dr. John Fernandez, at Nathan Littauer Hospital in Gloversville, who informed her that she had endometriosis as well as a pelvic infection. He recommended surgery. However, Dr. Fernandez wanted to wait to see if medication could clear up the problem so he decided to give her six months before he would operate. The six months passed, and Tonia's condition did not improve. In June, 1972, Dr. Fernandez operated on Tonia and removed her left ovary. The surgery was followed by hormone therapy, called Enovid-10, which prevented Tonia from having a regular menstrual cycle.

After several months of depression and ill health, Tonia finally started to feel strong enough to leave her sister. During those months, a strong urge to get her life in order began to emerge. She also began to feel a deep yearning to discover her own spirituality. Tonia had heard about the Zen Center in San Francisco where people learned to meditate and develop along the spiritual path. In the spring of 1973, Tonia thanked her sister and kissed her goodbye. She was off to San Francisco.

Once there she became friendly with a man who was practicing macrobiotics. Tonia had heard about macrobiotics and became interested in the diet and philosophy. Nevertheless, Tonia, whose ancestry is Puerto Rican, French, and Irish, was still attached to her mother's ethnic cooking. "And one of the things I loved was fried bananas," she says, laughing now through her words. "When I was told that if I wanted to practice macrobiotics correctly I would have to give up fried bananas, I said, 'Oh no, not that.' "

So Tonia ate brown rice, miso soup, and vegetables along with her dairy food, sugar, and fried bananas. It was then that Tonia decided to go off the Enovid-10 hormone treatment and never went back to it. Still, her health continued to deteriorate.

She stayed at the Zen Center for two years, meditating and studying Zen. After a while, however, she started to grow bored and wanted to have some fun.

Perhaps the devilish side of her started to awaken.

So Tonia quite the Zen Center and headed for the casinos of Lake Tahoe, Nevada, where she spent the next nine months "partying and drinking, day and night. I was having a great time," she says. "Looking back, though, I don't know how I ever survived that period in my life. All I did was gamble, party, and drink Scotch."

But the great time took its toll. Soon the pain in her abdomen became excruciating. "My periods became horrible. I was having a heavy flow, and a lot of vaginal discharge. I was feeling tense all the time and irritable. I was really getting sick."

Then the depression came back, and the party was over.

In April, 1976, Tonia decided to return east and settle in Boston, where she had friends and knew she could take care of herself. Within weeks after arriving in Boston, Tonia visited the South Boston Community Center where doctors diagnosed Tonia's condition as endometriosis and uterine cysts.

"My ovary had swelled almost to the size of a tennis ball," she says. In an effort to convince her of the severity of her condition, Tonia's physician pushed the ovary forward from within so that it bulged obscenely through her side. "It was really big," she relates.

Tonia's physician urged her to have an operation that would remove the ovary and perhaps the uterus, depending on what they saw once they opened her up. If the operation was performed, Tonia would of course lose any chance of having children again and would also have to undergo hormone therapy. Despite the hormones, however, she would begin to grow a lot of facial and body hair as a result of the loss of the female hormone, estrogen, which would be eliminated from her body with her ovaries.

Though she was very much afraid of what lay ahead of her, Tonia decided not to have the operation. She would wait. She had remembered that someone had told her that the macrobiotic diet could be effective against endometriosis. So she decided to try it. Goodbye fried bananas.

In May, she moved into a macrobiotic study house in Boston and ate a strict macrobiotic diet for a couple of months. However, as soon as she began eating only macrobiotic staples—whole grains, vegetables, various vegetable- and soybean-based soups and condiments—she suddenly became desperately ill.

"I was so fatigued that I could no longer hold down a job," Tonia says. "I was tired all the time." She developed this terrible "gnawing" inside, as if something were pulling on her intestines and sex organs from within.

She had now reached the nadir of her life: sick, tired, out of work, and depressed. Even macrobiotics didn't seem to be working. She thought about having the operation, and then she thought about all that facial and body hair and the fact that she would probably never live a normal life. She considered suicide.

And then fate seemed to intervene.

Jennifer Brown, a macrobiotic friend, offered to take Tonia in and provide food and cook for her until Tonia became well again. Jennifer cooked and supported Tonia for a couple of months. Slowly, her strength returned, and she began to feel better. When Tonia was strong enough Jennifer decided to move out of her apartment and Tonia assumed occupancy. In the summer of 1976, Tonia met Steve Gagne, whom she would eventually marry.

For the next year, Tonia worked at the East West Foundation, the educational organization dedicated to teaching macrobiotics, and continued to eat a wide macrobiotic diet. Her strength had returned, though she would occasionally go through bouts of fatigue. Also, the vaginal discharge continued, and she still suffered from occasional cramps.

At the time, Tonia was eating the standard macrobiotic diet, which includes whole grain flour products, fruit, oil, and small amounts of fish. Tonia wasn't sure how she was progressing but did not feel as if she were making great strides toward health.

In August, 1977, Tonia and Steve decided to have a consultation with Michio Kushi, president of the East West Foundation, at the organization's annual summer program in Amherst, Massachusetts.

"I sat down with Michio and he looked at my left hand and my left foot," she tells me. "He looked into my eyes and examined my face and then he said to me, 'You have no left ovary, right? Also, right ovary not so good, right? Also, tumor

111

in your descending colon.' Then he looked at me and said, 'Maybe you have cancer.' "

At this point, Kushi took out a piece of paper and drew a diagram describing in exact proportions what Tonia should be eating. He told her to eat 60 percent whole grains, the rest vegetables, miso soup, various condiments, and to avoid all animal products, especially dairy foods and meat. Kushi also told her to eliminate all oil, flour products, and fruit until the condition had been eliminated. He recommended that she take regular hip baths in daikon leaves, which he said would heal her sex organs. He also encouraged her to apply a plaster of taro potato over the area of her reproductive organs. She should do this regularly to help eliminate the implants on her sex organs, he said.

"Within two weeks after I followed that diet, the pain subsided. I had a feeling of elation. My energy came back and a lot of worry was gone," Tonia says.

After several weeks of progress, she seemed to have an occasional relapse. "I'd start to feel weak again, and then I would think about having the operation. But the relapses passed quickly and I would feel good again."

Although she seemed to make immediate progress on the healing diet Michio Kushi had given her, Tonia had to marshal every ounce of will within her to stick to it.

There were times when the cravings were overpowering and she had to have something outside the strict medicinal diet. Once she had a peanut butter cookie and another time a carob brownie, and both times, Tonia says, the symptoms of the endometriosis came back: pain, cramps, and "that gnawing feeling." Any small binge would immediately bring back the symptoms.

"I had to eat the limited diet Michio had given me for two years before I could assume a normal macrobiotic diet," she recalls. "Sometimes I would have to make desserts for Steve after we were married and I couldn't eat them. I used to go into the kitchen and cry."

Gradually, however, Tonia's taste for food began to change. Her cooking got better, and she learned to create dishes with grain and vegetables that simulated many of the foods she found herself craving. Soon she began to like the smell the food created in her house, and it wasn't long before she began to love the food. "I started to really appreciate the simple taste of macrobiotic food. Then I started to love the diet."

About seven months after she had begun the strict macrobiotic regimen, Tonia found out she was pregnant. "I was so happy, I was so grateful, that I wrote Michio Kushi a letter thanking him for everything, for my health, for this knowledge, for my child."

Six weeks after Tonia gave birth to Taran, she underwent a full examination by her physician which showed no signs of endometriosis. The disease was gone. And so were many other problems in her life.

Dr. Christiane Northrup, an obstetrician-gynecologist practicing in Portland, Maine, has requested that Nathan Littauer Hospital send her Tonia's records. So far, the records the hospital has provided Northrup are incomplete. However, based on the available information, Northrup stated that "Tonia's case is very unusual."

It is not surprising that Tonia's endometriosis came back in 1976 after she had had surgery five years earlier. "This is often the way the disease progresses," said Northrup. "It usually keeps getting worse," particularly if the person has stopped taking the hormone therapy, which Tonia had done. Without such therapy, there is no mitigating factor to keep the disease in check, and thus, "the symptoms continue to get worse, often to the point that a hysterectomy is needed," Northrup said.

In light of all of this, Northrup stated that Tonia's recovery "appears diet-related."

Today Tonia is trying to give back to others what she has been given. "I keep thinking what if people had withheld this information from me? Where would I be?"

Tonia and Steve Gagne, who is now director of the East West Foundation, give regular macrobiotic lectures and cooking classes in the Boston area as well as in other cities across the country. Tonia's once rebellious energy is channelled elsewhere now, and her relationship with her mother is one of love and respect.

In sharing her knowledge of food and health and in giving of herself, Tonia finds herself on the other side of the fence, helping others in need as she was once helped. "What I love most about it all is the simple gratitude people express. They sit down and eat a simple meal, and you watch them get better week by week; there's such a reward in sharing this knowledge with others and seeing it help them."

Yet, one need spend only a few minutes in Tonia's home to appreciate the center of her life—mothering. "Right now, my children are my life. But even when they're grown and gone, I always want my life to be one of nourishment for others."

EAST WEST FOUNDATION CENTERS

LISTING OF EAST WEST FOUNDATIONS AND AFFILIATES

The following East West Foundation offices have direct affiliation with the East West Foundation National Headquarters in Boston, Massachusetts. Each of these organizations offers regular counseling services, cooking classes, courses in macrobiotic philosophy and other macrobiotic educational activities.

National Headquarters:

Boston East West Foundation
17 Station Street
Brookline, MA 02147
(617) 731-0564

East West Foundation Offices:

Baltimore
4803 Yellowood Road
Baltimore, MD 21209
(301) 367-6655

Boston
17 Station Street
Brookline, MA 02147
(617) 731-0564

Philadelphia
606 South Ninth Street
Philadelphia, PA 19147
(215) 922-4567

Regional Affiliates:

California
708 N. Orange Grove Avenue
Hollywood, CA 90046
(213) 651-5491

Colorado
1931 Mapleton Avenue
Boulder, CO 80302
(303) 449-6754

Connecticut
184 East Main Street
Middletown, CT 06457
(203) 344-0090

Illinois
1574 Asbury Avenue
Evanston, IL 60201
(312) 328-6632

Washington, D.C.
P. O. Box 40012
Washington, DC 20016
(301) 897-8352

East West Foundation Medical Associates

The Medical Associates listed below may be contacted through the East West Foundation National Office, or through the affiliated centers listed on page 115.

Guillermo Asis, M.D.
Boston, MA

Keith Block, M.D.
Evanston, IL

Mr. & Mrs. Armando Diaz
Caracas, Venezuela

James P. Doyle, M.D.
Medical Director
Comprehensive Medical Servies
Newton Center, MA

George Elvove, M.D.
Chicago, IL

Fred Ettner, M.D.
Chicago, IL

Joseph A. Ierardi
Marlborough Hospital
Marlborough, MA

Otey Johnson, M.D.
Ardmore, OK

Edward Kass, M.D.
Channing Labs
Boston, MA

Alan Kenney, M.D.
Moncton, New Brunswick, Canada

Peter Klein, M.D.
Washington, D.C.

Haruo Kushi
Brookline, MA

Hy Lerner, M.D.
Phillipston, MA

Marilyn H. Light
Executive Director
Adrenal Metaboblic Research
Society of the
Hypoglycemia Foundation, Inc.
Troy, New York

Robert Mendelsohn, M.D.
Chicago, IL

Tatsuzo Nakamuro
Nishinomiya-city, Kyogo-ken
Japan

Dr. Yoshio Nomoto
Itami City, Japan

Christiane Northrup, M.D.
Milton, MA

Hideo Ohmori
c/o Nippon C.I. Foundation
Tokyo, Japan

Norman Ralston, D.V.M.
Dallas, TX

Kristen Schmidt, R.N.
Allston, MA

Mark Shusterman, M.D.
Boston, MA

John Sotiriou, M.D.
Rhodos, Greece

Richard J. Stephenson
American International Hospital
Chicago, IL

Tom Takase M.D.
Totigiken, Japan

Nicolo M. Tauraso, M.D., F.A.A.P.
The Gotach Center for Health
Frederick, MD

Dr. Chandrasekhar G. Thakkur
Sind Ayurvedic Pharmacy
Bombay, India

Mrs. Marion Tompson
President,
La Leche League International
Franklin Park, IL

Marc Van Cauwenberghe, M.D.
Boston, MA

Celso Vierira, M.D.
Ipanema, Rio de Janeiro
Brazil

Dr. Anthony Vincent, D.C.
Philadelphia, PA

David Wilson, M.D.
Oklahoma City, OK

H. Donald Won-Ken, D.O.
Waterville Osteopathic Hospital
Waterville, ME

Bibliography

Aihara, Cornelia, *Chico-San Cookbook,* Chico-San., Chico, CA.

Aihara, Cornelia, *The Do of Cooking,* 4 Vols., Ohsawa Foundation, Oroville, CA.

"An M.D. Who Conquered His Cancer," *Saturday Evening Post,*
     September, 1980, Indianapolis, IND.

Dufty, William, *Sugar Blues,* Warner Publications, New York, NY.

East West Foundation, *Cancer and Diet,* East West Publications, Brookline, MA.

East West Journal monthly, Brookline, MA.

Esko, Wendy, *Introducing Macrobiotic Cooking,* Japan Publications,
     New York, N.Y.

Esko, Edward and Wendy, *Macrobiotic Cooking for Everyone,* Ibid.

Kohler, Jean and Mary Alice, *Healing Miracles From Macrobiotics,* Parker
     Publishing, Englewood Cliffs, NJ.

Kushi Institute Study Guide bi-monthly, Kushi Institute, Brookline, MA.

Kushi, Aveline, *How to Cook with Miso,* Japan Publications, New York, NY.

Kushi, Michio, *The Book of Do-In,* Ibid.

Kushi, Michio, *The Book of Macrobiotics,* Ibid.

Kushi, Michio, *How To See Your Health: The Book of Oriental Diagnosis,* Ibid.

Kushi, Michio, *Natural Healing Through Macrobiotics,* Ibid.

Kushi, Michio, *Oriental Diagnosis,* Sunwheel Publications, London, England.

Kushi, Michio, *Visions of a New World: The Era of Humanity,*
     East West Journal, Brookline, MA.

Macrobiotic Case Histories, 7 Vols., East West Foundation, Brookline, MA.

Macrobiotic Review quarterly, East West Foundation, Baltimore, MD.

Mendelsohn, Robert S., *Confessions of A Medical Heretic,* Contemporary Books,
     Chicago, ILL.

Mendelsohn, Robert S., *Male Practice,* Contemporary Books, Chicago, ILL.

Ohsawa, Georges, *The Book of Judgement,* Ohsawa Foundation, Oroville, CA.

Ohsawa, Georges, *Cancer and the Philosophy of the Far East,* Swan House,
     Binghamton, NY.

Ohsawa, Georges, *Guidebook for Living,* Ohsawa Foundation, Oroville, CA.

Ohsawa, Georges, *Zen Macrobiotics,* Ibid.

Ohsawa, Lima, *The Art of Just Cooking,* Autumn Press, Brookline, MA.

Order of the Universe quarterly, Kushi Institute, Brookline, MA.

Sacks, Castelli, Donner and Kass, "Plasma Lipids and Lipoproteins in Vegetarians
     and Controls," *New England Journal of Medicine,* May 29, 1975,
     Boston, MA.

Sacks, Rosner and Kass, "Blood Pressure in Vegetarians," *American Journal of Medicine,* Vol. 100, No. 5, John Hopkins University, Baltimore, MD.

Select Committee on Nutrition and Human Needs, U.S. Senate, *Dietary Goals for the United States,* U.S. Government Printing Office, Washington, D.C.

Yamamoto, Shizuko, *Barefoot Shiatsu,* Japan Publications, New York, NY.

Notes on the Contributors

Keith Block, M.D. received his Bachelor of Science degree from the University of Florida and University of London in 1975. He graduated from the University of Miami School of Medicine in 1979, and participated in a one-year Residency Program at the Illinois Masonic Medical Center. Dr. Block is practicing privately in Evanston, Illinois, where he incorporates nutritional approaches in the care of variety of conditions. He has been practicing the macrobiotic way of life since 1975.

Marc Van Cauwenberghe, M.D. Received his medical degree from the University of Ghent in 1970. He served as medical editor of *Natural Healing through Macrobiotics* by Michio Kushi, published in 1978, and lectures regularly throughout Western Europe. He is currently in private practice in his native Belgium.

Peter Klein, M.D. graduated from LSU Medical School in 1972, and practiced a rotating internship at LAC-USC Medical Center. He conducted his first year psychiatry residency at Mt. Sinai Hospital in Los Angeles from 1973-4, and his second and third year residency at a UCLA veteran's hospital. He also received a fellowship in child psychology at Reis-Davis-USC Medical Center in 1976-77, and worked with the Los Angeles County Probation Department from 1977-79. He is the medical director of the Rica Regional Institute for Children and Adolescents in Rockville, Maryland. While Dr. Klein integrates the principles of macrobiotics, his medical practice is limited to the treatment of emotional and mental aspects of health.

Haruo Kushi received his B.A. from Amherst College in 1978. He is presently a doctoral student in the Department of Nutrition at the Harvard School of Public Health, and is participating with Frank Sacks, M.D. and associates at the Harvard School of Medicine in research dealing with the macrobiotic diet.

Michio Kushi was born in Kokawa, Wakayama-Ken, Japan in 1926. His early years were devoted to the study of international law at Tokyo University, and an active interest in world peace through world federal government in the period following the Second World War. In the course of pursuing these interests, he encountered Yukikazu Sakurazawa (known in the West as Georges Ohsawa), who had revised and reintroduced the principles of oriental medicine and philosophy under the name "macrobiotics". Inspired by Mr. Ohsawa's teaching, Mr. Kushi began his lifelong study of the application of traditional understanding to solving the problems of the modern world.

Mr. Kushi came to the United States 30 years ago to pursue graduate studies at Columbia University. Since that time he has lectured on oriental medicine, philosophy, culture and macrobiotics throughout North and South America, Europe and the Far East; he has also given numerous seminars on macrobiotics and oriental medicine for medical professionals and personal counseling for individuals and families, including many cancer patients. While establishing himself as the world's foremost authority on the macrobiotic approach, he has guided thousands of people to restore their physical, psychological and spiritual health and well-being as a fundamental means of achieving world peace. He has also presented an address to a special White House meeting and two addresses to the delegates of the United Nations on the applications of macrobiotic principles to world problems.

Mr. Kushi is founder and president of the East West Foundation, a federally-approved, non-profit, cultural and educational organization, established in Boston in 1972 to help develop and spread all aspects of the macrobiotic way of life through seminars, publications, research and other means. He is also the founder of Erewhon, Inc. the leading distributor of natural and macrobiotic foods in North America, and of the monthly *East West Journal* and the quarterly *Order of the Universe* periodicals. In 1978 Mr. and Mrs. Kushi founded the Michio Kushi Institute of Boston, an educational institution for the training of macrobiotic teachers and practitioners, with affiliates in London and Amsterdam; and at the same time, as a further means toward addressing world problems, established the annual Macrobiotic Congresses of North America and Western Europe.

Mr. Kushi's published works presently include *Natural Healing Through Macrobiotics, The Book of Macrobiotics, The Book of Do-in, How to See Your Health, Oriental Diagnosis, Visions of a New World: The Era of Humanity,* and the quarterly *Order of the Universe.* Mr. Kushi has presided at all the Foundation's Cancer Conferences; he presently resides in Brookline, Mass., with his wife Aveline and children.

Robert S. Mendelsohn, M.D. has served as Associate Professor, Department of Preventive Medicine, Abraham Lincoln School of Medicine, University of Illinois; Medical Director, American International Hospital, Zion, Illinois; and National Director, Medical Consulation Service, Project Head Start. He is a well-known author, through his nationally syndicated column *The People's Doctor* and his recent books *Confessions of a Medical Heretic* and *Male Practice.* One of the leading medical advocates for the macrobiotic approach, Dr. Mendelsohn had called for the inclusion of courses on macrobiotics and nutrition in medical schools, has authored introductions to several of Mr. Kushi's books, and has appeared at all of the Foundation's Cancer Conferences. Dr. Mendelsohn presently resides and practices in Chicago, Illinois.

Tom Monte, journalist, author, has worked as a staff writer for the Center for Science in the Public Interest in Washington, D.C. His story on Dr. Sattilaro's successful recovery from cancer through macrobiotics, *An M.D. Heals Himself of Cancer,* has appeared in the *East West Journal,* the *Denver Post* and other major newspapers, and the *Saturday Evening Post.* Mr. Monte is presently living in the Boston area, where he serves as an Associate Editor for the *East West Journal.*

Kristen Schmidt, R.N. received her A.A. Degree at the University of Cincinnati and her R.N. at the University of New Mexico in Albuquerque. From 1974-76, she worked as a staff nurse, specializing in labor and delivery, at Northwestern Memorial Hospital in Chicago. From 1976-80, she was a staff nurse, with a specialty in adolescent psychiatry and labor and delivery, at the University of Cincinnati General Hospital. She is presently working in private duty in Boston, and is completing advanced studies at the Kushi Institute.

INDEX

healing ability, natural, 18
hyperlipidemia, 54, 55
hypoglycemia, 85
hysterectomy, 23

I
insomnia, 96

K
kidney stones, 62
Kushi Institute, 8
Kushi, Haruo, 9, 63
Kushi, Michio, 7, 9, 11, 52

L
La Leche Legue, 49
Lemuel Shattuck Hospital, 8

M
macrobiotic diagnosis, 22-25
        dietary recommendations (see diet)
        way of life suggestions, 33-35
medical approach, diagnostic methods, 11
        failure of, 16,18
milk and milk products, 43,44
mucus, excess accumulation, 22-25, 55

N
National Cancer Institute, 51
nursing, 56-60

O
oil, cooking, 29
Oski, Dr. Frank, 44

P
pap smear, 48-50, 84, 85
plasters (see external treatments)
Pritikin Longevity Center, 73
protein, 16, 27, 43, 44
"Prudent Diet," 70, 71

R
reflections, daily, 5, 14

S
Sacks, Dr. Frank, 8
salt, 16, 29
Science News, 7, 14
Seelig, Dr. M, 44
soybean products, fermented, 46
sugar, 45
surgery, necessary cases, 18

T
taro plaster (see external treatments)
Taussig, Dr. H., 44
thrombosis, 100

V
valium, 48
vegetables, land, 28, 32
        sea, 28, 29, 32, 46, 47

W
water, 16
White House, macrobiotic presentation at, 52

X
x-rays, 51